Community
Health Concepts & Issues

Ameliorative
dichotomy

Community Health Concepts & Issues

Richard Wigley

James R. Cook

Eastern Illinois University

D. Van Nostrand Company

New York • Cincinnati • Toronto • London • Melbourne

Cover photographs:
Top left: Industrial pollution *(Free Lance Photographers Guild)*
Top right: Prosthetic valve operation *(Courtesy of the World Health Organi-zation)*
Bottom left: Medical research *(Courtesy of Eli Lilly and Company)*
Bottom right: Health counseling *(Courtesy of the World Health Organiza-tion)*

D. Van Nostrand Company Regional Offices:
New York • Cincinnati •

D. Van Nostrand Company International Offices:
London • Toronto • Melbourne

Library of Congress Catalog Card Number: 74–20381
ISBN: 0–442–21633–5

Published by D. VAN NOSTRAND COMPANY
135 West 50th Street, New York, N. Y. 10020

10 9 8 7 6 5 4

Preface

Community Health: Concepts and Issues presents a comprehensive overview of the field and of the professional community health worker, whose role has become increasingly important in the face of the complexities of today's health problems. In light of its recent emergence as a major influence in the health sciences, community health requires an approach that goes beyond the traditional textbook structure. We have designed this book not only to describe the basic philosophy and concepts of the field but also to give the reader insights into the issues, controversies, and challenges in a growing profession charged with the responsibility of controlling these problems.

The book is intended for students in an introductory course in community and public health. Most students come to the course with varied backgrounds, interests, and classroom exposure to the health sciences. Because community health work and research in recent years have been undertaken in other professions, such as sociology, psychology, and political science, students in these disciplines are often exposed to the basic philosophy and methodology of community health. We have therefore written this book both for students in the health sciences and for those in other disciplines to whom its contents would be of value in performing their academic and occupational tasks.

The book is divided into three parts. Part One deals with the nature of today's major health problems. The dramatic shift in the health patterns of recent decades from acute-communicable to chronic-degenerative diseases has been accompanied by a growing awareness of the importance of behavioral characteristics—habits and life styles—in the cause, treatment, and prevention of many of our serious diseases. Our primary concern in this section has been to provide a framework within which current health problems can be described and studied in light of these behavioral influences.

Part Two outlines the particular methods and techniques by which the community health worker identifies and measures the scope and intensity of health problems. New methods and techniques, some of which are based on trial and error, are often difficult to develop and implement because of the multiplicity of factors that affect such major health problems as pollution, drug abuse, heart disease, and cancer.

Part Three is concerned with the organization and procedures by which health care is delivered to the consumer by the community health profession. As health needs have become increasingly difficult to meet, the community health worker has played an increasingly significant role in our contemporary programs of health care delivery and research. This section discusses the organizational problems of the health profession that hinder effective and efficient delivery of health care and the recent innovations that have been proposed and implemented to help solve these problems.

Contents

8. Community Health Education   164

Utilization of Health Services
Compulsory vs. Voluntary Participation
Determinants of Health Behavior
Summary
References
Suggested Projects

9. The Dilemma of Health Care Delivery   186

Precipitators of the Crisis
Inequities in Health Care
The Cost Explosion
Quality of Care
The Organizational Solution
References
Suggested Projects

10. Innovations in the Health Field   208

Financing Medical Care
From Private Practice to HMOs
Surgi-Centers: A Solution to Costs
Comprehensive Health Planning: Toward Better
*   Organization*
Consumerism: A New Force in the Health Field
Medical Manpower: Meeting the Demand
Summary
References
Suggested Projects

Index   237

Part One

The Status of Contemporary Health Problems

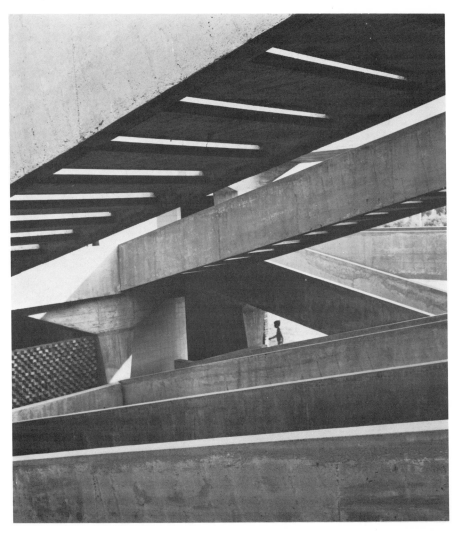

"Buildings should be modern, of course, but should not be out of scale with man as a social animal."—Dr. Robert-Henri Hazeman, Inspecteur Général of public health in France. *(Photo on previous page courtesy of the World Health Organization)*

1. Introduction

Community health is an ever-changing and evolving field; it varies according to time and place. Our study of community health will examine it in its most modern form.

Contemporary community health must be understood in terms both of "community" and of "health," for a multitude of factors related to each contributes to the eventual decisions that produce the programs designed for the health maintenance of the population. The community and the health field interact, resulting in conflict as well as cooperation; what seems advantageous and desirable to one segment may appear needless and even deleterious to the other. An understanding of the nature of this interaction and of the complex of factors operating on it is essential to successful community health work. The starting point for this understanding is the knowledge of what, in a contemporary sense, is meant by the terms "community" and "health."

WHAT IS COMMUNITY HEALTH?

Historically, "health" was measured primarily in physical terms and was defined objectively as the absence of disease. Today, reflecting basic changes in the types of dominant health problems, health is measured in terms of mental and social, as well as physical, well-being, and the judgment of health is often subjective, individual, and relative. From the contemporary viewpoint, health involves the complete individual functioning as a whole within his cultural and physical environments.

In earlier times, "community" was fairly easy to identify in terms of health problems and their solutions. Before the turn of this century, communicable diseases were the major health threat throughout the world. Since communities were generally more isolated from one another then than they are today, infectious diseases were often confined naturally to the specific community where the outbreak occurred, and, even in severe cases, quarantine measures could often be effectively initiated in a community to stop the threat of spreading to the outside. Providing a health service was thus usually a matter of dealing with an isolated problem in a well-defined area. In general, the political and geographical designations of a community—town, city, county, and so on—sufficed to identify a community for health purposes.

Quite a different picture of the community confronts the health professionals today. Americans are a highly mobile population whose communities are not necessarily restricted by political and geographical boundaries. A community is defined wherever the needs of an individual are being met. To secure a service or purchase an item, the individual crosses county, state, and even national boundaries, and in so doing he sets new boundaries of his community. The contemporary individual thus has many communities to which he belongs.

In much the same way, contemporary health needs and problems may involve a neighborhood, an ethnic group, a town, county, several towns or cities, or an entire state or country. Water pollution in one town may be affecting not only that community but several towns upstream where refuse is being dumped into the nearby river. Air pollution may afflict many cities in a large geographical area. In meeting the demands for medical services, contemporary health planners often must consider more than the politically defined community and realize that the "community" involved in a particular health problem may be a multi-county or multi-city area. Moreover, in some instances the "community" may be defined in terms of a special group of people, such as the aged, blacks, or children. In each case, the community varies both with the population being dealt with and the problem to be solved.

The clear identification of not only the health problem but also the "community" affected by it is essential to effective health programming. Demographic data such as age, sex, religion, ethnic group, socioeconomic status, educational background, and occupation are important in this identification of a community for health purposes. For example, sickle-cell anemia is a problem affecting only a certain segment of the total population. Special medical attention and educational programs should therefore be directed at this particular segment. Similarly, many other health needs and problems affect a single segment within the total population, and programs should be geared to this group.

Realizing the increasing diversity of health needs and the consequent problem of community identification to meet such needs, the National Commission on Community Health Services in 1966 developed the concept of *community of solution* as a guide to the planning and development of community health programs. Figure 1.1 illustrates the idea that the delivery of community health services must reflect the fact that health problems can involve populations and geographical groupings different from those established by the usual political and geographical boundaries. Consequently, the *community of solution* comprises the geographical area(s) or group(s) of people that must be approached to solve an existing health problem.

The community-of-solution concept offers the advantages of

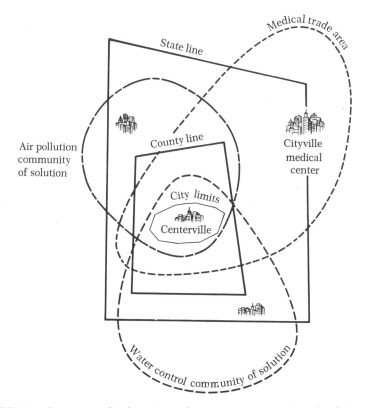

FIGURE 1.1. One geographical area may have many communities of solution. Political boundaries, shown in solid lines, seldom cover all of a community's health problems or medical trade areas. *(From* Health Is a Community Affair; *a report of the National Commission on Community Health Services. Cambridge: Harvard University Press, 1966, p. 3)*

more efficient use of resources, more effective health care delivery, and more cooperation among all health professions. A single county health department with a relatively small population base, for example, may lack the financial resources to develop health services that require certain specialties and expensive equipment. Reviewing its needs, this department might find it advantageous to combine with a neighboring health department to form a multi-county unit with a larger population base and greater financial and professional resources. Similarly, two or more small communities may combine their financial resources to build a centrally located hospital to provide health care to an area encompassing several political jurisdictions. Here again, the problem to be solved dictates the "community" to be defined and helped.

With the increasing diversity of our health problems and the greater mobility of our population, the community-of-solution concept seems better suited as a guide to defining and solving problem areas than the traditional adherence to political and geographical boundary lines. Health professionals continually face the challenge of planning better and more efficient health programs, and the correct identification of the area and population to be approached is essential in meeting this challenge successfully. Through this concept, needless programs can be tabled and, more importantly, short-sighted, ineffectual programs dealing with only half the problem can be better avoided.

AN HISTORICAL PERSPECTIVE

Mankind has always believed in a better place where life is free of stress and toil and where health and happiness abound. For some it has been an Arcadian setting in the remote past; for others it is a utopian dream of the future. Yet history suggests that struggle is synonymous with life and the idyllic dream of Paradise may not be compatible with the evolution and survival of man. Every civilization, whether primitive or advanced, has been fraught with problems that detract from the "good life." Even the glorified Polynesian who appeared to Captain Cook as the epitome of health and happiness suffered from the elements of primitive life, not the least of which were human sacrifice, social stratification, and a variety of diseases. Illness and disease are coexistent with life, and ancient man like modern suffered from a myriad of problems. Consequently, always dreaming of a better life and in reality confronted with constant adversity, man has been forced to devise a complex network of elements to protect and promote the health of the individual and the group. In its modern form we may call this the practice of community health.

Cultural forces have shaped the development of community health practices. Factors which determine a society's attitude toward life—such as religion, philosophy, and social and economic conditions—exert a controlling influence on the institutions, practices, and procedures of health care in that society. Health-keeping practices do not operate in a vacuum, but are an integral part of the total sociocultural system, and they can be understood only within the context of the society in which they function. Health practices reflect the idiosyncrasies of each culture, and many health care procedures may be functional only within the particular society where they are practiced. This fact holds true whether we consider primitive man driving out evil spirits through rites and incantations or modern specialists attempting chemotherapy on a leukemia victim.

Health practices have existed since the beginning of man. Although the first written accounts of medical practice are found in

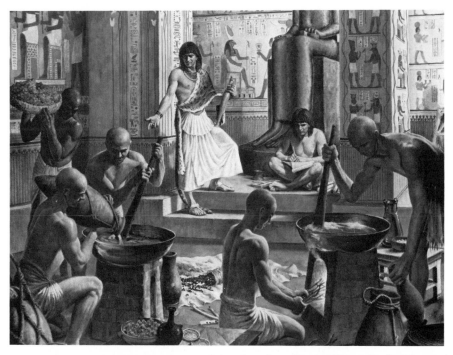

Egypt, c. 1500 B.C. Although Egyptian medicine dates from about 2900 B.C., the best-known and most important pharmaceutical record is the *Papyrus Ebers* (1500 B.C.), a collection of 800 prescriptions mentioning 700 drugs. Egyptian pharmacists were priests who learned and practiced their arts in the temple. *(Courtesy of Parke, Davis & Company, © 1957)*

Egyptian papyri dating from around 1900 B.C., the knowledge, beliefs, and practices they describe are the obvious accumulation of many centuries of humanity: centuries through which man lived, survived many ailments, populated the earth, and achieved social and technological advances—all without benefit of the "germ theory" of disease or the ensuing medical advances of recent times.*
Furthermore, despite the recent progress in medical expertise and technology in American and Western European cultures, Western medicine has few better remedies for many common ailments than did the Greeks 2,500 years ago. In fact, many of the doctrines of Hippocrates when put into modern medical jargon would sound like those of any modern physician attempting treatment of the common cold or arthritis. Even modern programs in public health are built upon ideas centuries old. In the Book of Leviticus there is a written hygienic code which deals, as Hanlon has summarized, "with a wide variety of personal and community responsibilities, including cleanliness of the body, protection against the spread of contagious diseases, isolation of lepers, disinfection of dwellings following illness, sanitation of campsites, disposal of excreta and refuse, protection of water and food supplies, and the hygiene of maternity."[1] In like manner the Romans preceded the twentieth century in much of the engineering achievements which have provided modern advances in sanitation. Even today some of the original drainage systems of the Romans are still in use, having been incorporated into the present-day sewage systems of Rome. Thus, although many current health practices are indeed advanced, they are not without precedent.

Even definitions of health and disease are not absolute, but rather reflect cultural values and attitudes. Within American society it would be difficult to obtain a consensus on the meaning of health. Some people tolerate minor ailments without any thought of being ill, while others seek medication for nonexistent problems. As A. L. Knutson remarked: "The line between wellness, malingering, and illness is in good part a socially drawn line. Aches and pains that are not experienced as out of the ordinary for oneself and one's social colleagues may not be perceived as illness."[2] Consequently, Americans accept obesity, poor eyesight, and the common cold as readily as some primitive cultures accept infestation with intestinal

---

* The "germ theory" maintains that diseases are the result of specific organisms invading the body. *Specific etiology,* or the study of these specific organisms (usually microbial) which cause disease, has been the major foundation of medical theory and practice in Western societies throughout most of this century.

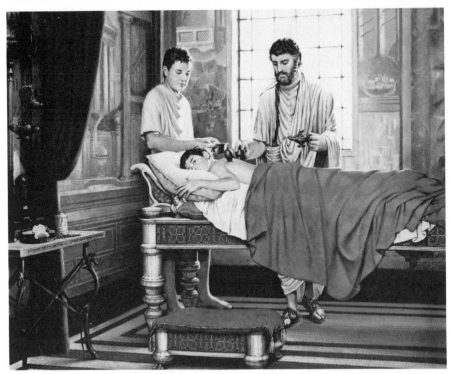

Rome, c. 170 A.D. A Greek himself, Galen (130–200 A.D.) was a physician to Roman emperors and commoners. He is considered the last important practitioner in the millennium of Greek domination of the medical world, and his teachings were accepted as dogma for fifteen hundred years. Cupping was one of the forms of treatment he advocated. *(Courtesy of Parke, Davis & Company, © 1958)*

parasites. Few people are overly concerned about the colossal business being done by the psychiatric profession in America, and it is quite likely that future generations will wonder at our indiscriminate use of antibiotics and other chemicals which may carry unforeseen consequences. But our community health practices, as is true of all cultures, reflect attitudes and value judgments which are not necessarily objective or scientific yet nonetheless exert a major influence on the health care system of the nation.

In a given time and place, community health programs reflect the interaction of three elements: (1) the nature and severity of health problems, (2) theories on cause, cure, and prevention and (3) the prevailing social ideologies of the period.[3] As an illustration of (1), an epidemic disease, killing thousands of people, will elicit more drastic health measures than one that develops insidiously over a period of time, slowly increasing debility but offering no immediate threat to life. Similarly, a patient who is told that he will die within twenty-four hours without his medication will show a higher level of motivation to take that medication than will the heavy smoker to stop smoking though he is told that he may develop heart disease or cancer in the distant future by continued smoking.

It is now a matter of record that the crippling effects of polio, although affecting a relatively small number of people, prompted an expensive and intensive research program which culminated in preventive measures and which had the full support of the general public. More recently, phenylketonuria, a poorly understood cause of mental retardation affecting only about one person in ten thousand, has prompted at least forty-one states to enact laws requiring that newborns be tested for the problem even though the tests and treatments are not well proven. In both of these diseases, the population affected (small children) and the severity of the outcome have been the major determinants of the programs developed.

The current research emphasis in America on cancer, heart disease, and stroke reflects the importance of these ailments in a society that has largely controlled the epidemic diseases and has an increasing population in the age group most affected by these conditions. By contrast, in many underdeveloped countries where the largest percentage of the population dies at an early age from communicable disease or malnutrition, there is little need for elaborate programs in the prevention of heart disease. Similarly, to the plague-ridden communities of fourteenth-century Europe, concern over death from cancer was negligible. Each of these examples illustrates how health programs reflect the nature and severity of existing health problems in a particular place and time.

Also important to the development of health programs are the theories on cause, cure, and prevention. Medical cures and illness prevention are inevitably based on a theory of causation, whether it be an imbalance of elements in the human body, as in the *humoral theory*,** or the presence of a specific pathogen as identified in the germ theory. In the Hippocratic treatise *Airs, Waters and Places,* climate is considered a major factor in disease, and special consideration is also given to the life style of the people, nutrition, and the surrounding physical environment. Community health programs based on this theory would vary significantly from those of the early twentieth century in America when the search for the microbial agents of disease dominated efforts to cure and prevent

---

** The *humoral theory* states that there are four humors, or elements, in man—blood, phlegm, yellow bile, and black bile—and that a person is healthy when these humors are mixed in the proper proportions and ill when this balance is upset.

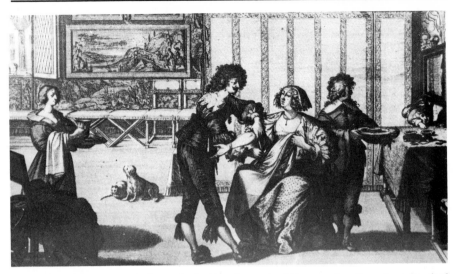

France, c. 1650 A.D. The charlatans in the French courts of the seventeenth century, laughed at by Molière, used cure-alls that had not changed since Galen: purges, bleeding, and cupping. A king of France was purged 2,000 times and was bled 38 times. He lived to be 77. *(Courtesy of the World Health Organization)*

illness. Similarly, the fact that theories on the cause of a problem directly reflect what is done to eliminate or ameliorate the condition can be easily seen in current approaches to heart disease. Because it is believed that a major type of heart disease is caused by the excessive accumulation of fats in coronary arteries, health personnel encourage low-cholesterol diets, emphasize jogging for physical fitness, and emphatically condemn cigarettes in an effort to prevent or control the build-up of fats. These measures are still based on a theory, however, and although much advanced, it is like those of centuries ago in maintaining an element of conjecture in its formulation. For Western medicine, the danger lies not in the theories but in the belief of their absolute truth. Such blind faith often breeds an uncritical attitude toward the medical procedures based on these theories. Man must constantly review and evaluate his basic theories in view of the impact they have on his total community health.

The final interacting element which plays a role in community health programs is the prevailing social ideology of the society. Health programs and practices cannot be separated from the religious and philosophic assumptions or the political organization and economy of a given group. The Social Darwinism of the nineteenth century, which considered society to be governed by laws of nature leading to the survival of the "fittest," would foster a different approach to community health than do the humanitarian feelings of our present society. An underprivileged person would have little chance for adequate health care in nineteenth-century America as described by Dobzhansky:

> In cities of nineteenth-century Europe and America poverty and squalor persisted cheek by jowl with mounting comfort and luxury. . . . Most of mankind became "subject races," to be uplifted and perhaps even civilized; the pedagogic method was to put the subjects to work for the profit of their white masters. If some of the latter felt a need to put their consciences at rest, a church hymn solved the problem:
> > The rich man in his castle, the poor man at his gate
> > God made them high and lowly.
> > He ordered their estate.[4]

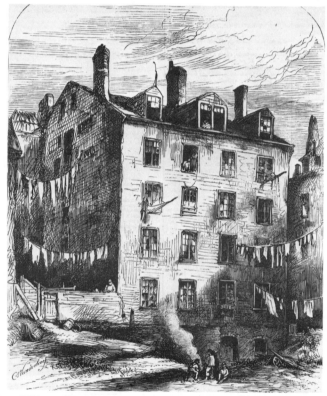

United States, 1871 A.D. Health measures for the poor in mid-nineteenth-century America were generally ineffectual, ignored, or, most likely, nonexistent. In keeping with the prevailing ideology of separate "estates" for the rich man and the poor man, little was done to eradicate the poverty and filth that created and perpetuated the spread of disease and infection among the lower classes. The above tenement house in Mulberry Street in New York City was condemned by the New York Board of Health in 1871, and then reoccupied in 1873. *(National Library of Medicine, Bethesda, Maryland)*

This period held little hope for the poor and oppressed, and even health programs reflected the belief that the existing conditions of poverty and ill-health would ensure, on the part of the poor, a respect for superiors and gratitude to Providence for the blessings they did receive.

Comparing this ideology with current attitudes toward health care, one can see the obvious effect of differing values on the kinds of programs being pursued. Health is now considered a basic right of all Americans; the value we place on human life forces our medical profession to save the deformed child, prolong the life of terminal patients, and decry attitudes favoring euthanasia. Similarly, as beliefs in the desirability of children and the positive experience of parenthood are juxtaposed with attitudes favoring population control, the paradoxical situation is created in America whereby researchers are designing techniques to increase the fertility of some, while large research funds are spent discovering ways to limit the fertility of others.

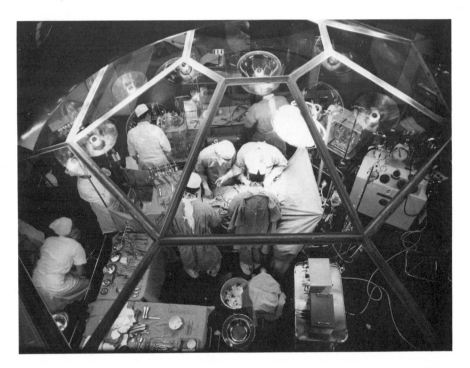

Medicine today. The rapidly expanding technology in twentieth-century Western societies has not only made possible organ transplants and survival by machines long after death would "naturally" have occurred, but has also all but eliminated diseases that were the major causes of debility and death not even a half a century ago. A major question facing man today is whether his social growth will be able to keep pace with his scientific advancements. *(Courtesy of the World Health Organization)*

It is axiomatic that history never catches up with the present and that the present is always one step behind the future. However, in our era of technology and rapid change, the elements of past, present, and future fuse so quickly as to become nearly indistinguishable. From the first airplane to the first man on the moon, from insulin to kidney machines, has been but a short step in time. Consider the astronaut and the medical doctor whose elementary teachers told them that space travel and organ transplants would never be possible. What are the implications for the community health profession of the fact that the medical doctor and his elementary teacher are only a generation apart? That books on folk medicine and space medicine can be read with near-equal popularity? That acupuncture and cryogenic techniques can be performed in the same hospital?

In an era of penicillin, plastic surgery, and pacemakers, is there anything to be gained from a study of historical ideas and concepts? Is there any value in studying today's health problems and programs as reflections of the same underlying considerations—severity of disease, theories of causation and prevention, and societal ideologies—that affected the past? When newness and unprecedented events are the order of the day, can history offer anything of value to the community health professional in his effort to understand, if not control, the health problems of the day?

SUMMARY

In one form or another, community health activities are as old as man himself. Although today's health programs are more elaborate and complex, they are influenced by the same forces as those of centuries ago. To arrive at a clear understanding of contemporary community health, the health professional must be aware of these underlying forces which continue to shape his approaches and which make health programs relative according to time, place, and need. Failure to understand this relativity can result in short-sighted approaches to problems that are obviously temporary in light of the constantly changing health needs of a population. In viewing current community health practices from an historical perspective, the health professional should become more aware of forces which shape health programs and therefore more constructively critical of programs for which he might be responsible. We can learn from the past, and what has gone before us can provide a salient perspective for the future.

REFERENCES

1. John J. Hanlon, *Principles of Public Health Administration,* 5th ed. (St. Louis: C. V. Mosby Co., 1969), p. 15.
2. Andie L. Knutson, *The Individual, Society, and Health Behavior* (New York: Russell Sage Foundation, 1965), p. 48.
3. Lenor S. Goerke and Ernest L. Stebbins, *Mustard's Introduction to Public Health,* 5th ed. (New York: Macmillan Co., 1968), p. 4.
4. Theodasius Dobzhansky, *Mankind Evolving* (New Haven: Yale University Press, 1962), pp. 10–11.

TOPICS FOR DISCUSSION

1. Explain the concept of "community of solution." Use several examples to show how this concept is functional in solving health problems.
2. How has the concept of health changed in recent times? Explain how this might affect the field of community health.
3. Analyze a current health program (cancer research, multiple sclerosis program, and so on) in view of the three basic interacting factors described in the chapter.
4. List and discuss some modern theories about health and disease which may prove totally false in future years.
5. Discuss some of the ancient theories about health which seem to be ludicrous today. Analyze these theories with respect to the basic understanding of man and the universe prevalent at that particular time.

2. The Nature of Contemporary Health Problems

Diseases most prevalent in modern industrialized nations also afflicted prehistoric man and exist today in all primitive societies; diseases have unchangeable and universal characters because man's nature has remained essentially the same for some 100,000 years. The relative prevalence of the various diseases, however, has changed from one historical period to another and differs today among geographical areas and social groups. Differences in the total environment and in the ways of life make for this diversity.[1]

Within the twentieth century the developed countries of the world have experienced a radical change in the types of health problems affecting their populations.* The transition began in the early nineteenth century with public health measures designed to improve living conditions through sanitation, personal hygiene, and better housing. Soon thereafter the bacteriological work of Louis Pasteur, Robert Koch, and others was to result in the germ theory of disease. The combination of these early public health measures with the concept of specific etiology precipitated an unprecedented era of communicable disease control. Prior to the twentieth century, infectious and contagious diseases were the major causes of illness and death in the United States. By reviewing Table 2.1 it can be readily seen that from 1900 to the present, the leading causes of

---

* The material in this chapter deals with the nature of health problems in the United States and similar industrialized nations. This is not to deny, however, the worldwide importance of many health problems which at present are well controlled in the United States.

16

death in the United States have radically changed. With minor variations, this chart would hold true for most of the developed countries of the world that have the benefit of Western medical techniques, proper nutrition, and adequate sanitation. It should be noted, however, that this table reflects causes of death and in no way indicates the amount or types of health problems which, while not causing death, exact a heavy toll of personal debility, economic loss, and family hardship.

As can be seen, the acute communicable diseases have declined as leading causes of death and those of a degenerative nature have increased. In addition, evidence shows that mental illness, drug abuse, and certain ailments of affluence (obesity, pollution, and accidents, for example) pose serious health threats in modern societies. Many of these current health problems are not really new, though their magnitude and importance are perhaps unprecedented, yet it is exactly these problems which are the least understood. They deny easy adherence to the specific-etiology concept, which seeks to identify the specific agent causing a particular disease and which is so fundamental in the control of communicable diseases. Like all health problems, but perhaps to a greater degree, the health concerns of contemporary societies are intricately woven into the fiber of each society's values and life styles. Consequently, the assessment of social factors is germane to a clear understanding of these health problems.

TABLE 2.1   Leading causes of death per 100,000 population, United States, 1900 and 1970*

	1900			1970	
Rank	Cause of death	Rate	Rank	Cause of death	Rate
1	Influenza and pneumonia	202.2	1	Heart disease	360.9
2	Tuberculosis, all forms	194.4	2	Cancer	162.3
3	Gastroenteritis	142.7	3	Cerebrovascular	
4	Diseases of heart	137.4		disease (stroke)	101.6
5	Cerebrovascular disease		4	Accidents	56.2
	(stroke)	106.9	5	Pneumonia	29.0
6	Chronic nephritis	81.0	6	Diabetes mellitus	18.8
7	All accidents	72.3	7	Arteriosclerosis	15.5
8	Cancer	64.0	8	Cirrhosis of liver	15.4
9	Certain diseases of		9	Suicide	11.5
	early infancy†	62.6	10	Homicide	8.3
10	Diphtheria	40.3		All causes	942.6
	All causes	1,719.1			

* From the National Center for Health Statistics
† Birth injuries, asphyxia, infections of newborn, etc.

VENEREAL DISEASE AND SOCIETY

Health problems, whether a communicable disease such as cholera or a degenerative problem such as lung cancer, cannot be diagnosed out of the context of the environmental setting in which they occur. In 1943 it was demonstrated that penicillin was highly effective in the treatment of venereal disease, and public health leaders were confident that the control of both syphilis and gonorrhea was imminent. But, as Figure 2.1 illustrates, their optimism was ill-founded. The incidence of syphilis and gonorrhea showed an initial decline when penicillin first began to be administered, but since the late 1950s it has been steadily rising. Gonorrhea is currently the number-one reportable communicable disease in the United States. Many experts maintain that the disease has reached epidemic proportions, and it shows no signs of abating. How do we account for this "epidemic"? To begin with, we must go beyond the specific-etiology concept and understand that the ability of a virus or bacterium to reach and overtake the host is dramatically affected by various characteristics of the society and people involved.

Researchers, epidemiologists, doctors, and public health offi-

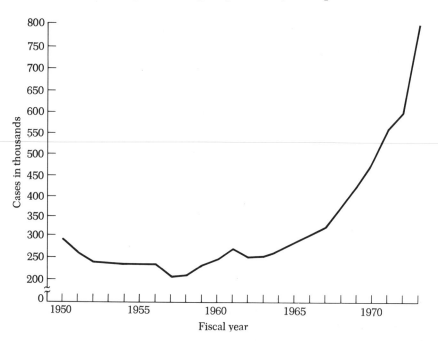

FIGURE 2.1.   Reported cases of gonorrhea per 100,000 population, by year: United States, 1950–1973. *(Reproduced with permission of Technical Information Services, Bureau of State Services, Center for Disease Control, Department of Health, Education, and Welfare)*

cials can offer myriad reasons for the increase in the incidence of venereal disease, and generally these reasons reflect the influence of social elements. Much blame has been placed on the birth control pill since it eliminated the fear of pregnancy and, so the reasoning goes, thus increased sexual activity among the young. Yet sociological research does not substantiate this view; rather it indicates that we have experienced an increasing liberalization in sexual behavior since the late 1920s and the pill has not suddenly altered the sexual activity of the young.[2] It should be noted, however, that the availability and use of the pill has decreased the use of the condom which served as both a contraceptive device and a somewhat effective venereal disease preventive. This fact, rather than promiscuity, probably reflects the true impact of the pill on rising venereal disease rates.

The real point, however, is still to be considered. The use of contraceptive devices and our sexual values are part of contemporary American society, and if they do, in fact, have an effect on venereal disease incidence, then society's role must be analyzed.

The increasing liberalization of sexual values is mirrored in the mass media. Sexuality is exploited at every turn, being used to sell everything from cars to toothpaste. Erotic messages are ubiquitous. Basic institutions and long-standing rules are being actively questioned. While technology appears to create a cold, impersonal world, people seek refuge in the warmth of close personal relationships. The pleasure of the moment seems more certain and important than the dubious future. In this atmosphere there is greater emphasis on individual choice in sexual matters with less absolute control exerted by outside forces.

But a paradox exists. For all of this liberalization, society still views venereal disease in a disapproving fashion reminiscent of the days when it was considered a retribution for a sexual sin. Thus, society provides the setting for greater sexual freedom and, concomitantly, more venereal disease, while eliciting the shame and guilt in many who contract the disease which prevents them from seeking prompt treatment.

In a more specific way the cause of the current gonorrhea "epidemic" reflects this influence of the society. Having an incubation period of three to five days, gonorrhea becomes communicable very quickly; couple this fact with the jet-age mobility of Americans and the possibility exists for the rapid spread of gonorrhea over large areas. A disease contracted in New York can be carried to Los Angeles in a few hours. Additional problems are created when victims are ashamed of having the disease and fail to report the problem or try to "protect" their contacts by refusing to give their names.

Thus, the current rise in venereal disease incidence is the result of a complex of factors, many of which are social in nature. Realization of this fact is extremely important since it helps dispel the naive view that in communicable diseases the only necessary elements are a causative agent and a susceptible host. It is clear that social factors are important considerations in the study of communicable disease, and it is necessary to recognize that much of what is considered *elimination* of a disease by medical techniques may simply be *control* due to such factors as a better standard of living and proper nutrition.

This control-versus-elimination concept is readily demonstrated in the case of polio. Following the development of the polio vaccine, the incidence of polio declined rapidly and people began to believe that the disease had been eradicated. This naive view led many parents to become lax in the immunization of their children. The result is a currently large number of nonimmune children who are now susceptible to polio. Public health officials fear an epidemic of polio if one active case is introduced into an area where high numbers of such children reside.

Similarly, there have been some recent cases of typhoid fever reported in Florida, Texas, and several areas in Mexico. This disease also has been controlled in the past through vaccination and, most importantly, through good sanitation. As the disease became controlled, however, people again relaxed their vaccination schedules and sanitation procedures. Under such conditions the disease is likely to present a problem once again.

In both of these instances, the disease has not been eliminated, only controlled. It is up to health officials and individuals to keep in check those factors which can precipitate a resurgence of the diseases.

SOCIAL ETIOLOGY OF CHRONIC DISEASES

If social factors are of paramount importance in the causation of communicable diseases, how influential must they be in health problems where a single communicable cause is not discernible and where a complex of possible causative factors merge to produce illness? The answer is obvious and the message even more so: in the etiology of contemporary health problems, social factors are dominant, and a clear understanding of these factors is requisite to the development of adequate health programs.

The veracity of the preceding statement is most vividly exemplified in an analysis of the two biggest killers in America: heart disease and cancer. Rather than revealing a specific causative agent, studies of these diseases indicate a group of *contributing* factors which play a role in their causation.

Research on heart disease points to the sedentary life style of Americans as a precursor of early arterial degeneration, and early heart attack victims are notoriously unfit. Similarly, dietary habits (particularly a high intake of saturated fats), cigarette smoking, emotional stress, and overweight have been implicated in the development of heart and circulatory problems. Each of these items is closely tied with the life styles and values of a society whose "good life" involves, physiologically, maximum intake with minimum output. Under these circumstances effective action against heart disease involves the identification and alteration of those elements which foster individual behavior conducive to the development of heart problems. The individual must have the motivation and understanding to produce preventive behavior which extends over a lifetime.

In a similar manner, cancer, especially certain types, has shown a dramatic increase in recent times, with much of the problem attributable to sociocultural factors. Historically, this relationship

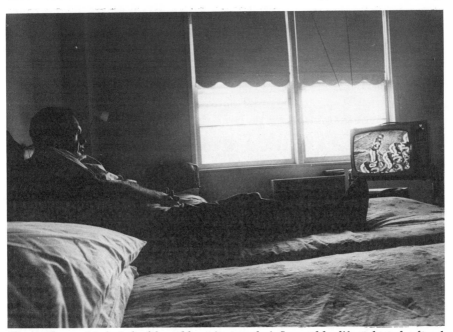

The incidence of today's health problems is strongly influenced by life style and cultural values. The sedentary way of life of many Americans, especially those in highly urbanized communities, has been implicated directly in the development of heart disease, America's number-one cause of death. *(Courtesy of the World Health Organization)*

between cancer incidence and the social environment is documented in the incidence of scrotal cancer among chimney sweeps in eighteenth-century England. In their book on medical sociology, Freeman, Levine, and Reeder describe the problem as follows:

> Scrotal cancer was peculiarly characteristic to chimney sweeps in eighteenth century England. The train of events leading to contraction of scrotal cancer, as Sir Percival Pott found in studying the disease in 1775, was somewhat as follows: (1) an environmental need for heated dwellings (2) was met with a sociocultural response in the form of widespread installation of home space-heaters (3) the preferred fuel for which produced so much smoke and soot that (4) exhaust passages required frequent cleaning; (5) an occupation, chimney sweep, developed which put the worker into close and frequent contact with soot which caused scrotal cancer.[3]

A more recent example involves the incidence of lung cancer in the American population. In 1914 only 371 deaths due to lung cancer were reported in the United States. By 1930 the number was 2,355 and in 1968 there were 55,300 deaths due to lung cancer. The overwhelming evidence points to cigarette smoking as a leading contributor to this increase, and the death curve for lung cancer closely parallels the smoking curve for the nation during this period.

Although experts disagree as to the exact role of cigarettes or the causative mechanism involved, there are few medical researchers who would deny that there is a definite link between cigarette smoking and lung cancer. Yet this popular habit has become a major part of the life style of many Americans, and the actual discomforts of stopping smoking seem to outweigh the potential dangers of continued smoking, especially for a population which emphasizes the present.

Analysis of the total situation shows that several elements in combination have led to the increase in cigarette consumption. Dr. Hal Levine, Chief of the Pulmonary Disease section at Hines Hospital in Chicago and a leading crusader against cigarette smoking, has given an interesting review of the social acceptance of the cigarette.[4] According to Levine, cigarette smoking was considered effeminate at the beginning of the century, and "real men" chewed tobacco and subsequently spat in the ubiquitous spittoons of the period. Also during this period tuberculosis was the leading cause of death, and soon a connection was made between the spread of the Tubercle Bacillus and the frequent expectorations of "chewers."

With the mass production of an aseptic looking little "number" all neatly rolled and packaged, the stage was set for the popularization of the cigarette and smoking soon became the masculine thing to do—even to the point that women were excluded. Shortly, however, the economic-minded tobacco industry realized that it was missing half the market and, as Levine points out, there has been a recent campaign to encourage women to smoke. Utilizing the current emphasis on women's liberation, smoking advertisements have pushed the cigarette as an obvious indicator that "you've come a long way, baby." Similarly for the male, the masculine emphasis is still dominant and to "light up" is considered a "cool" thing to do.

One further example of societal influence in contemporary health problems can be found in the increasing problem of ulcers. For some time now, observers and researchers have argued that psychological and social factors are influential in the causation of peptic ulcers. Interestingly, a major change in the pattern of this illness has occurred in this century in western Europe, Scandinavia, and the English-speaking countries. Before the 1900s, more females than males suffered from the ailment, but today many more males than females are afflicted. Physiologically, no change has apparently occurred in males and females, but there have been many changes in sex roles as well as in family structure. Similarly, there are variations of this affliction relative to class, with mortality from duodenal ulcers highest among the highest socioeconomic class. An investigation of the influence of social factors on this physiological disorder would no doubt contribute to a better understanding of ulcers, their treatment, and prevention.

AFFLUENCE AND AFFLICTION

At this point, we have had only a partial view of contemporary health problems, for the problems of alcoholism, drug addiction, mental illness, psychosomatic illness, accidents, and pollution head a long list of conditions which seem to plague the industrialized nations of the world. In its own way, each of these problems detracts both from the overall quality of health in the population and from the total wealth and effectiveness of the society. The actual magnitude of these problems is staggering, the causes are many, and the cures, at this point, are mostly conjecture. In these problems, however, the influence of social factors is clearer at least, even though poorly understood and often inaccurately assessed.

In recent times, volumes have been written analyzing the social etiology involved in each of these problems. Such factors as poverty, alienation, stress, anxiety, and rapid change have all been cited.

Many authorities differ over the dominant factor in these ills, but generally the concept which emerges from their studies is that man is a complex, integrated organism functioning in a similarly integrated environment and, therefore, that his diseases can be precipitated by subtle and insidious alterations in this integration. For instance, professional literature in sociology and medicine is filled with studies on the stress of modern living and its link with a host of physiological and psychological disorders. Stress, however, is different things to different people. Further, the inherent and developed capacities of the individual to deal adequately with stress will determine its ultimate effect. Consequently, each individual problem is unique and reflects a particular combination of influencing factors which make it essential to know both the nature of the disease and the nature of the patient in order to effect adequate treatment.

This concept of stress and its impact on modern man is clearly expressed in Alvin Toffler's book *Future Shock.* Although not identifying specifically with the term *stress,* Toffler's main thesis is that the rapidity of change in technological societies is outrunning man's adaptive powers and thus creating both psychological and physiological trauma. To add credence to this theory, Toffler cites

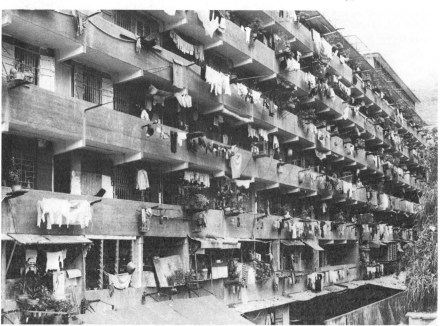

Overloading the environment with stresses from too much noise and pollution and overcrowding force many people beyond their ability to cope. The poor in modern societies are often the hardest hit; conditions of poverty, crowding, and unemployment often characterize the background to drug use. *(Courtesy of the World Health Organization)*

the research of Dr. Thomas H. Holmes and Richard Rahe who designed a research tool to measure the amount of change occurring in an individual's life in a given span of time.

In gathering their data, the researchers were interested in a variety of changes in the lives of their subjects. They asked about job changes, vacations, divorces, deaths, births, financial crises, illness, change in diet, and any element which would cause a change or produce trauma in the individual's life. Utilizing this Life-Change Unit Scale, Holmes and Rahe began to compare the "life change scores" of thousands of individuals with the medical histories of these people.

> And seldom were the results of an experiment less ambiguous. In the United States and Japan, among servicemen and civilians, among pregnant women and the families of leukemia victims, among college athletes and retirees, the same striking pattern was present: those with high life change scores were more likely than their fellows to be ill in the following year. For the first time, it was possible to show in dramatic form that the rate of change in a person's life—his pace of life—is closely tied to the state of his health.[5]

Thus, the impact of numerous life changes, especially dramatic ones, seems to be linked to physiological breakdown. Perhaps it is true, as many authorities warn, that it is impossible rapidly to introduce considerable change or novelty into a society without simultaneously causing imbalances in the population's body chemistry. Each time we introduce a new scientific and technological entity we may be placing biologically one more adaptive burden on ourselves.

If change affects us physiologically, what must its psychological impact be on the human organism? With experiences, people, situations, ideas, information, and attitudes rapidly bombarding the neural systems of people in changing environments, the answer is all too obvious—man has overwhelmed his mental adaptiveness and finds himself in confusion and disorientation. The increased use of drugs, the apathetic and hopeless responses of millons, the increasing vandalism and violence, and the constant search for meaning in a seemingly meaningless world are evidence of the above state of affairs. Further, it seems that much of mankind has passed beyond the limit of individual decision-making in response to the overwhelming numbers of choices available.

Man, like all other animals, has an "adaptive range" within which he is capable of physiologically and psychologically coping with the change and novelty present in his environment. Change below or above this range can have negative effects on the total organism. Each individual is different in terms of this adaptive range, but everyone has a potential "breaking point" in terms of physiological and psychological stress. To exemplify this concept, one has only to look at tactics used in concentration camps to "break" prisoners. Both solitary confinement, in which the prisoner receives no sensory input, and constant, round-the-clock questioning under bright lights, offensive voices, and real or threatened physical torture, are sufficient to cause psychological breakdown. In everyday life this principle is most apparent in relation to over-stimulation of the senses in which the overloading of the environment with stresses—such as noise, chemical pollutants, and crowded quarters—is taking a bulk of Americans beyond their adaptive range.

The mental illness, alcoholism, and drug addiction so prevalent

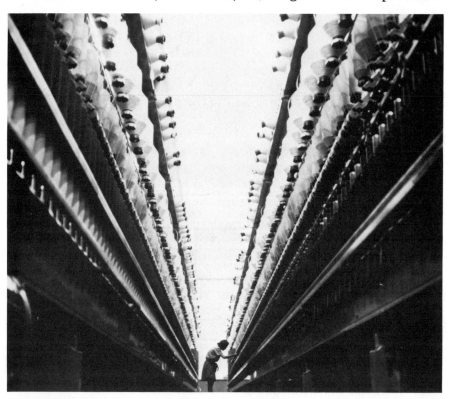

Although occupational accidents, afflicting one worker in ten in industrially developed nations, constitute a major health problem, there are other occupational hazards in such countries: the soul-destroying monotony and stresses of modern production methods with their assembly lines and shift work. Inside this modern textile plant, highly automated processes put a heavy strain on the remaining employees whose work companions are machines and not human beings. *(Courtesy of the World Health Organization)*

at this time may only reflect a basic orientation of society, and programs designed to solve these ills must begin at the causes of them. It is difficult to understand how an aspirin-popping, caffeine-gulping, martini-sipping culture that makes such behavior not only glamorous but a sign of adulthood could help but spawn addictive disorders in its population, especially when that society increasingly presses in on the individual with its technology and, in so doing, may be creating fewer and fewer opportunities for self-identity and personal fulfillment. How does the individual develop security in a ghetto slum? Are the pressures of marketing deadlines and bureaucratic red-tape conducive to self-fullfillment? Where is the personal satisfaction for the assembly-line worker who has no feeling for and often never sees the product of his work? The answers to these questions would point to conditions that create personal frustrations whose outlet is often a chemical euphoria—the harbinger of drug addiction and alcoholism.

Yet the genesis of such problems is often misunderstood. Late in 1973 it became legal for nineteen-year-olds to drink in Illinois. During the debate on this volatile issue, opponents of the bill voiced the opinion that the law would increase "problem" drinking in Illinois. It is naive to believe that alcoholics are legislated into being, and such a view reflects a poor overall assessment of this health problem.

The dimensions of the health problems discussed in this section are great; they accurately reflect the social turmoil in technological countries. The solutions to these problems will be difficult, but without a clear understanding of their genesis we will waste our efforts at amelioration. In assessing these problems and in effecting adequate programs, health professionals should keep the following concept clearly in mind.

> Social and technological achievements have spread economic affluence, increased comfort, accelerated transportation, and controlled certain forms of disease. But the material satisfactions thus made possible have not added much to happiness or to the significance of life. Not even the medical sciences have fulfilled their promises. While they have done much in the prevention and treatment of a few specific diseases, they have so far failed to increase true longevity or to create positive health. The age of affluence, technological marvels, and medical miracles is paradoxically the age of chronic ailments, of anxiety, and even of despair. Existentialist nausea has found its home in the most affluent and technologically advanced parts of the world.[6]

MULTIPLE CAUSATION AND A WORKABLE MODEL

In keeping with the complex nature of contemporary health problems which by now should be evident, the idea of multiple causation must replace the older idea of specific etiology. Health problems must be analyzed for the causative influence of physical, mental, and social elements, and efforts must be made at a correct assessment of the interdependence of such elements in the development of contemporary health problems. The exact opposite of the specific-etiology concept, the concept of multiple causation is an attempt to view this interrelationship from a broad ecological base whereby man is seen as a functioning organism within a total environment. With this concept it will be possible to develop a feasible perspective through which man can more accurately assess the nature of his problems.

To arrive at this perspective, it may prove helpful to think in terms of basic needs of man and then view some consequences if these needs are not met. In essence, this need/problem model is as follows:

Needs of man	*Problems if needs are not met*
I. Food, Air, Water	I. Deficiencies or Excesses
II. Proper Use and Care, Sleep, Rest, Relaxation	II. Constitutional or Degenerative Ailments
III. Ego-preservation and Enhancement	III. Mental Disorders
IV. Absence or Control of Pathogens	IV. Communicable Diseases
V. Absence or Control of Excessive Forces	V. Traumatic Illnesses

I. Food, Air, Water. Adequate and appropriate ingestion of foods in the proper combinations and quantities, including all of the essential nutrients, water, and roughage, and the inhalation of pure air for necessary oxygen are requirements for the survival of the organism. If these requirements are not met, malnutrition, deficiency diseases, or nutritional excesses or "perversions" may occur. (The term "perversion" is used to include ingestion, inhalation, or injection of harmful drugs, nicotine, tars, or the consumption of excessive amounts of particular substances such as alcohol or dirt.)

II. Proper Use and Care, Sleep, Rest, Relaxation. This section identifies the needs for physiological expression and functioning for optimal growth and development. These include sleep, rest, exercise, relaxation, recreation, and the routines of personal hygiene. This latter subgroup of needs consists of the natural requirements for cleanliness as well as the learned and acquired needs resulting from socializing processes in group living. The larger category further includes the need for professional medical care and supervision when something goes wrong in order to prevent excessive damage or an increase in the degenerative rate. If these needs are not met, constitutional (malfunctioning of body parts) and degenerative (wearing out of body parts) illnesses, diseases, or defects may occur.

III. Ego-preservation and Enhancement. The needs for the development, preservation, and enhancement of the ego are included here. Self-identify, personal esteem, and self-fulfillment are basic requirements for the mental health and stability of the individual. These needs have both positive and negative aspects. The individual requires protection from undue stress, but at the same time he must be exposed to stressful situations in order to learn how to deal with stress. (Both internal and external stresses are implied here.) If these needs are not met, functional (psychologically induced) disorders, neuroses, or psychoses result.

IV. Absence or Control of Pathogens. This category represents the need for preventing pathogenic organisms from invading body tissues, organs, or systems. In practice this need is met by keeping pathogens away from the human host or by controlling or preventing their success in causing disease once an invasion occurs. If this need is not met, communicable or infectious diseases occur.

V. Absence or Control of Excessive Forces. The need for preventing body tissue collision or contact with excessive physical or chemical forces is represented in this final group of needs. There are many forces existing in the environment which humans cannot tolerate in an unfavorable encounter. These include impact with objects as large as automobiles or as small as bullets or radiation particles. They also include extremes in heat or cold, chemical poisons, allergens, strong electrical currents, submersion in liquids, or inhalation of a host of gases, fumes, fogs, smog, mists, and so on. If this need for protection is not met, traumatic illnesses such as shock, injuries, and poisonings can occur.

These five categories of health needs and resulting problems if the needs are not met are broad enough to encompass all that is known to be required for optimum growth, development, and functioning. All illnesses known to medical science, when their specific causative mechanism(s) is (are) identified, fit into one or more of the broad problem categories.

These needs remain constant throughout the life cycle of man from the moment of conception until death. The intensity of certain specific requirements may vary for an individual from one stage in development to another, or from one individual to another in the same developmental stage. But the needs themselves remain constant. Similarly, the threat of certain types of problems may be greater in one category than another, or for individuals in different age groups, or for certain individuals within the same age group. But the threat is constant throughout the life cycle.

From this model the concept of multiple causation can be readily exemplified. Take the case of a man suffering from cirrhosis of the liver. This ailment falls under need/problem category II. But the problem is the result of excessive alcohol intake and poor nutrition which reflect need/problem category I. Still, the heavy alcohol consumption may stem from inferiority feelings, failure, or various other psychological problems which are part of need/problem area

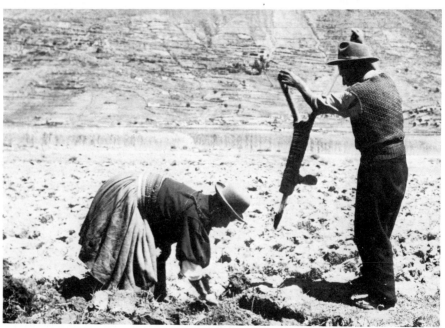

In contrast with its incidence in technological societies, hypertension is rare among the people of the high Andes. An hereditary factor is no doubt operating. Life at 14,000 feet, generation after generation, seems to encourage the development of the blood vessels in number and strength, thus improving the circulation and giving greater tolerance to conditions of high altitudes. *(Courtesy of the World Health Organization)*

III. Clearly, then, this problem is the result of several factors occurring in combination, and treatment of the problem must be directed at each of the causative factors. In a similar manner, many contemporary health problems could be adequately analyzed in view of this need/problem paradigm.

One further point must be emphasized concerning the causation of health problems. It is always important to realize that there are certain foundations or factors which determine and set limits to the health potential of everyone, individually and collectively. First, there is the genetic past (species and racial) and the current (individual) mixture of genes existing within each of us. The significance of genetic factors in problems ranging from alcoholism and schizophrenia to heart disease and cancer is still under study, and many researchers are convinced that an important connection does exist.

Secondly, the physical (air, climate, geography) and social (class structure, education) environments to a large extent determine the health status of the individual. The iodized salt so common in American stores reflects the discovery that simple goiter was common in those localities where iodine was not prevalent in the diet and thus exemplifies the geographical influence on health status. Similarly, as we have already seen, elements in the social environment have a significant effect on health concerns ranging from diet to medical treatment.

Finally, health status is reflected in both the overt behavior and inner feelings of the individual in response to his physical and social environments. This phenomenon is most easily observed in the triggering of physiological responses by psychological mechanisms—such as embarrassment leading to blushing or anxiety producing an increase in digestive juices.

So once again the point is reinforced: health problems—especially those of contemporary technological societies—are the result of multiple factors occurring in combination, and the understanding of this multiplicity is the essential foundation of effective health programming.

AN OUNCE OF PREVENTION

As health problems change, so do—or should—the programs designed to ameliorate them. And as modern industrialized nations attempt to deal with their contemporary maladies, the most fundamental change in future health programming will come in the increasing emphasis on preventive, rather than curative, measures. The reasons behind the emphasis on prevention are many, and a review of some of them will demonstrate the necessity of this shift.

As any fan of American Western movies can tell you, a person with the "fever" or some similar affliction would be banned from entering towns in the Old West. Similar techniques of ostracism were effective in Biblical times to control leprosy. The carriers of epidemic diseases were a direct threat to other people, and such measures against individuals seemed justified in light of the possible consequences to the total community. Such urgency or obvious outcome from a failure to respond immediately are not characteristic of ailments like heart disease, cancer, and ulcers, which develop slowly and generally are a threat only to the individual himself in some distant time. Yet they are the kinds of chronic ailments which last for long periods of time, usually cause much debility, and often require constant treatment. These characteristics coupled with the increased cost of medical care make the treatment of such problems economically devastating and emphasize the need for prevention. The acute short-term nature of infectious diseases allowed the luxury of waiting for crises to occur and then doing what you could when they did, with the understanding that shortly the infected person would either recover or die. The availability, cost and nature of current health treatment preclude such a crisis orientation and necessitate health programs that foster preventive measures in the community.

Emphasis should also be placed on the rehabilitation of those afflicted so that they can be returned to societal usefulness. It is personally beneficial and socially positive for individuals to be able, if at all possible, to contribute their part to the group. At present, efforts in this direction are being made through special education programs, drug and alcohol rehabilitation, physical therapy, and social programs for the aged and handicapped. Recent efforts to rehabilitate the mentally ill within the community setting rather than isolate them in far-off institutions mirrors this changing philosophy.

Contemporary health problems require new approaches which will help ensure both length and quality of life resulting in personal satisfaction and worth. Future programs to meet this end must be based on the realization that given the nature of current health problems, prevention and rehabilitation must replace the archaic crisis/intervention approach characteristic of times past. Indeed, an ounce of prevention may be worth a pound of cure, and rehabilitation may transform uselessness into social worth and personal dignity.

SUMMARY

Health problems reflect both time and place, and one can learn much about a culture by reviewing its health problems. Currently, the developed countries of the world have learned to control—not eradicate—many of the microbial diseases which continue to plague the underdeveloped countries. This success, however, has created new problems that require somewhat different approaches to their solution. The germ theory of disease, based on the identification of a single specific cause, does not prove adequate in dealing with problems that are multiply caused.

The concept of multiple causation requires that researchers analyze the total setting in which a health problem occurs. Problems such as heart disease, ulcers, drug addiction, and even many communicable diseases are often caused by many factors, and they require close analysis to understand this complexity. From such analyses we can obtain a clearer perspective on the nature of these health problems as well as devise more effective treatments of them.

The present state of community health can best be described as complex, transitory, and fragmented, and there is little doubt that the entire field will undergo many drastic alterations in the next two decades or so. This upheaval is not unlike that which many of our institutions are presently experiencing as a result of numerous and complex changes in the composition of the population and in the way people live. It is the result of changing disease patterns and of the rapid expansion of medical knowledge. It represents greater public awareness of health problems and the demand for better, more efficient and economical health care. It is the reflection of a general sense of frustration in the face of health problems for which immediate and convenient solutions are not available. In general, so many medical and social changes have occurred so rapidly in the past two decades that the transition from conventional and obsolete to creative and comprehensive health programs has yet to be successfully accomplished.

To understand the present challenges to the community health profession is to understand, insofar as possible, the complex social and medical problems that have emerged or been intensified over the past few decades.

The purpose of this chapter has been to provide an overview of the nature of health problems facing modern industrialized nations. Special emphasis has been placed on the concept of social etiology, since this concept may prove to be the major point of departure in future efforts at the solution of these health problems. The purpose of the following two chapters is to present a brief overview of the current status of today's major health problems as classified in the model presented in this chapter. The coverage of each problem area is not complete and no attempt has been made to discuss all their ramifications; rather the intent has been to provide a frame of reference within which the problems and functions of community health can be studied.

REFERENCES

1. René Dubos, *Man, Medicine and Environment* (New York: Frederick A. Praeger, Inc., 1968), pp. 76–77.
2. Phillip Cutright, "The Teenage Sexual Revolution and the Myth of an Abstinent Past," in *Family Planning Perspectives* (January 1972), pp. 24–31.
3. Howard E. Freeman, Sol Levine, and Leo G. Reeder, *Handbook of Medical Sociology* (Englewood Cliffs, N.J.: Prentice-Hall, Inc., 1963), p. 71.
4. From an address by Dr. Hal Levine presented in Springfield, Illinois, in April 1970.
5. Alvin Toffler, *Future Shock* (New York: Random House, 1970), p. 293.
6. René Dubos, *So Human an Animal* (New York: Charles Scribner's Sons, 1968), p. 14.

TOPICS FOR DISCUSSION

1. How have the health problems of the United States changed during the twentieth century? What are some basic reasons for this change?
2. Give some reasons for the current increase in venereal disease.
3. What does it mean to say that communicable diseases are controlled rather than eradicated?
4. Explain the Life-Change Unit Scale and its significance for the health field.
5. Why is the prevention of health problems even more important today than it was in earlier times?
6. Take several health problems and identify their basic cause. Then pursue them further and develop a view of them as multiply caused, identifying as many contributing factors as possible.
7. Do an historical analysis of some dread disease such as the plague. Look specifically for influencing social conditions of the

time and discuss the reasons for the periodic epidemics and then recessions of the disease.

8. Using a problem from the communicable disease group and one from the chronic-degenerative group, discuss the following statement: "Health problems cannot be understood out of the social and cultural setting in which they occur."

3. Communicable and Noncommunicable Diseases

COMMUNICABLE DISEASES

When the medical history of the twentieth century is written, undoubtedly the first half of the century will be identified as one of the most important periods in the entire history of medicine. The sciences of microbiology, pharmacology, and sanitary engineering combined forces to provide the ways and means for a full-scale attack on the leading killers of the day, the infectious diseases. The result was a dramatic reduction in the mortality rate from these acute diseases and a corresponding increase in the number of people who survived the crisis years of infancy and childhood. While some communicable diseases, such as venereal disease and hepatitis, remain major medical problems, the severe threat of specific infectious agents to the general population has, from a medical point of view, been reduced to a nuisance factor.

A nuisance factor in medical terms, however, is far from insignificant in the day-to-day problems of the health consumer and the medical practitioner. Infectious diseases continue to be a major source of depletion of energy, finances, and time to millions of people in this country. To the normally healthy segments of the population, no other single classification of disease causes more lost working hours, absenteeism from school, and expenditures for medical services and products than communicable diseases. Internists and general practitioners devote approximately half of their time treating infectious diseases and write more prescriptions for these conditions than for any other health problem. In 1973 Americans spent over 500 million dollars for cold remedies alone. The total "bill" is over 3 billion dollars a year—a high price to pay for a nuisance factor that in most instances will "run its course" regardless of the treatment given.

Despite the relative security of the present control over major communicable diseases, there is a developing concern among microbiologists that new and severe health problems of a communicable nature are beginning to occur. It should be of no great surprise in this era of ecological concern that these problems result from the application of the very pharmacological discoveries to which major credit was given for the control of pathogenic diseases. The abundant use of vaccines and antibiotics has apparently produced high levels of resistance to these medications in some organisms and has upset the ecological equilibrium of others. Within the past few years evidence has emerged to indicate potentially dangerous disease conditions arising from both the emergence of drug-resistant strains of pathogens and the development of conditions called super-infections, which result from biological disturbances in man's internal ecology.

Drug-resistant Pathogens

For many years now a great deal has been said about the overuse of antibiotics for the treatment of infectious diseases. Current medical literature continues to document the use of antibiotics not only as a curative for bacterial diseases—the proper use of antibiotics— but also as a preventative for potential bacterial infections. Viral diseases in which treatment with antibiotics is contraindicated are often treated with antibiotics on the assumption that secondary bacterial infections, such as bronchitis and bacterial pneumonia, will be prevented. Many hospitals as a matter of course administer antibiotics before all surgery in order to decrease the possibility of infections occurring during postoperative recovery. Combined with the curative use of antibiotics, these practices have resulted in such a prolific administration of such drugs that in 1972, for example, the amount of antibiotics administered was equal to 50 single doses for every person in the United States. To provide indicated treatment for microbial diseases for every person in the United States, this amount would be sufficient for a five-year period.

The predictable result is that some pathogens are beginning to develop strains that are resistant to specific antibiotics in varying degrees. Most strains of syphilis and gonorrhea are still fully curable by penicillin, but the amount and potency of the drug necessary to cure them has steadily increased over the past 15 years. Administration of the drug must therefore be spread over a longer period of time, thereby increasing the span of communicability of these diseases.

The control of typhoid fever in the United States has been threatened by the emergence in Mexico of a strain of typhoid bacillus which is resistant to previously effective antibiotics. These drugs have been sold without prescription in Mexico for a number of years, and their widespread use has apparently resulted in the development of resistant bacterial strains. The threat of a return to prominence of typhoid fever in the United States as a result of the organism being brought in by carriers is very real.

Super-infections

Among the many environmental problems resulting from ecological imbalances, perhaps the least publicized are those related to microbial organisms. The internal environment of man is an ecosystem, populated by large numbers and varieties of organisms living in either symbiotic or parasitic relationships and dependent upon each other for the maintenance of a suitable environment for reproduction and survival. Occasionally, virulent pathogens will enter the body from the outside or existing forms will overreproduce and cause the symptoms of infectious disease to occur. Antibiotics may then be administered to destroy the pathogens and cure the disease. Occasionally, the antibiotic destroys additional bacteria or otherwise upsets the microbial ecosystem in such a way that formerly harmless bacteria may become pathogenic and cause disease.

Although the extent of disease complications resulting from super-infections is unknown, there is evidence to indicate that relapses of certain infectious diseases are so caused. In addition, it has been estimated that as many as 100,000 cases of gram negative septacemia (a severe form of blood poisoning) are a result of super-infections. Fatalities from this condition have been estimated to be as high as 30,000 per year.

The Problem of Attitude and Health Behavior

Perhaps the most significant problem related to infectious diseases is not their occurrence but the development of a pattern of public attitudes and behaviors related to the medical treatment of all diseases. The public view of how diseases should be treated is strongly influenced by the treatment patterns used in the control of communicable diseases.

The elimination of the infectious diseases as threats to life has produced profound changes in both the nature and complexity of the health problems which confront contemporary society. On a superficial level, communicable diseases have been viewed by all but the medically sophisticated as simple cause-and-effect conditions in which the human body is violated by an unseen but externally produced organism. "Catching" a disease, therefore, was perceived as an unfortunate accident of nature over which a person had no control. The perceived simplicity of these diseases is reflected in our methods of prevention, treatment, and control—all of which are mechanistic, routine procedures requiring little individual effort beyond an occasional immunization, antibiotic treatment, and "two aspirin and rest in bed."

While our life span is longer and potentially more productive in the absence of severe infectious diseases, there is a certain irony in the simplistic behaviors and attitudes which our battle with these diseases has produced. There seems little doubt that contemporary health problems are in part a product of these earlier experiences. The search for simple explanations and the dependence on outside sources—such as doctors and medications—for the solution to health problems not only result in prolonged neglect of chronic diseases but are fruitless in the face of those problems which are products of complex social, psychological, and chemical processes and are deeply ingrained in our life styles. Where are the simple cause-and-effect relationships in alcoholism, mental stress, obesity, drug abuse, pollution, heart disease, and cancer? What doctor or hospital can we go to for a quick and easy cure? How often have you heard: "If we have the technology to send men to the moon, why can't we clean up our environment?" or, "If we can transplant organs, why can't we cure cancer, alcoholism, drug addiction?"

We have had our day of simple answers and complete reliance on outside sources for solutions to our health problems. We are now dealing with habits of living, customs, ways of life. No longer will the crisis-oriented attacks on disease processes be adequate to thwart the advances of health problems for which man, more than nature, is responsible. Certainly, the medical and health sciences will continue to add to our understanding of disease processes, but until the day comes (and hopefully it never will) when every movement and thought of the human organism is programmed, our control over the severe problems of the day will depend upon individual adaptability to the pressures and stresses of our life style and each individual's personal willingness to assume the responsibility for contributing to a quality existence for all.

CHRONIC DISEASES

Most of today's major health problems of a physical origin are *chronic* diseases. Such diseases are characterized by a gradual emergence and continuance of clinical symptoms over a period of months or years or by the varying and periodic occurrence of symptoms. Cancer is an example of a chronic disease in which symptoms develop over an extended period of time; arthritis is a chronic disease often characterized by periods of weeks or months when symptoms disappear, though eventually they return. In contrast to chronic conditions, *acute* diseases produce symptoms within a matter of days or weeks and reach their height of severity quickly. Most communicable diseases are acute in nature.

Taken together, the chronic diseases constitute today's number-one disease and medical care problem. One of every six persons is chronically ill, and more than two-thirds of all deaths in this country are due to chronic illnesses. Since length of affliction and prolonged medical care are major characteristics of chronic diseases, their rapidly increasing incidence has an enormous effect on present and future health care needs. Most of today's hospitals have inadequate facilities for extended care and, where they do, the cost is often prohibitive to the poor and elderly. The need for continual treatment is producing a disproportionate burden on already overworked doctors, nurses, and social workers. The spiraling costs of medical care are further inflated by the emerging technology in the treatment and rehabilitation of the chronically ill.

A further element in the cost of chronic diseases is reflected in lost productivity and income from diseases which strike during the productive years. A common misconception about chronic diseases is that they are confined mainly to the elderly. As shown in Figure 3.1, however, disability from these diseases is common at all age levels. Further evidence indicates that over half of those with chronic illnesses and two-fifths of the invalids are between the ages of 15 and 64 and more than one-third of the chronic invalids are under the age of 45. Diseases such as cerebral palsy, rheumatic heart disease, rheumatoid arthritis, diabetes, multiple sclerosis, and muscular dystrophy all have their onset before the period of old age. Cancer and heart diseases, although occurring predominantly in middle and old age, are distributed to varying extents in all other age groups. For each age group, the loss from chronic diseases of years of productivity, happiness, and contributions to society is enormous.

Degenerative Diseases

The human organism is a fantastically complicated "machine" that operates with a capacity and efficiency unequalled by any other animate or inanimate form of existence. Like other "machines," however, human organisms are subject to breakdowns and inefficiencies brought on by constant use and/or abuse of their parts.

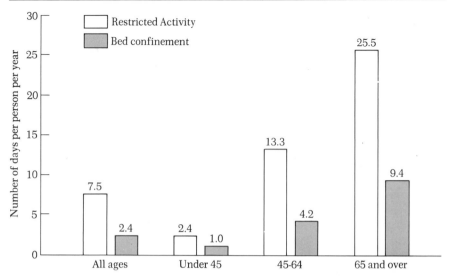

FIGURE 3.1. **Average number of disability days due to chronic diseases, by age: United States, 1972.** *(National Center for Health Statistics, U.S. Public Health Service)*

Tissue degeneration is a basic characteristic of all living things. In humans, "wear and tear" on body tissues and organs produced by normal physiological functioning over a period of years or by improper care of the body can result in inefficient operation of body systems, a condition generally referred to as a degenerative disease. Cardiovascular diseases and arthritis are common examples.

Over 70 percent of all deaths in this country are due to degenerative diseases, with heart and circulatory diseases being the predominant causes of death. The emergence of degenerative diseases as such serious problems in this country is due primarily to successful control of those diseases fatal in infancy and the early years of life. The obvious result has been an increase in the number of persons surviving the early years and living long enough to be affected by the degenerative process. Life expectancy at birth has increased from 50 years in 1900 to approximately 71 years at present. For this reason there is some justification in the view that the overwhelming incidence of degenerative diseases in this country is the sign of a "healthy" population and of effective methods of disease control and treatment. This statement, however, is limited to the degenerative disease rate that occurs among the elderly and belies the most crucial problem with degenerative diseases—the increasing incidence among those in the young and middle-age groups.

Cardiovascular Disease. A cardiovascular disease is broadly identified as any condition that interferes with the efficient circulation of blood through the body. So defined, the term covers a multitude of possible conditions from heart attacks to varicose veins to congenital heart defects. Those that are caused by degeneration, however, are fewer in number but occur much more frequently than those that may have a different etiology. Degenerative cardiovascular diseases most commonly result from deficiencies in the vascular system—blood and blood vessels—rather than in the heart muscle itself. If the blood is not flowing properly through the vessels to meet the nutrient needs of body cells, then the heart must pump faster and harder to force a sufficient amount of blood to body tissues. This additional work by the heart speeds up the degenerative process until gradually it becomes unable to pump sufficient amounts of blood. A usually fatal condition commonly called "heart failure" or "heart congestion" results.

Vascular problems are commonly caused by the following conditions: (1) arteriosclerosis, or hardening of the arteries, usually resulting from a combination of mineral deposits built up gradually in the walls of the blood vessels and a weakening of arterial muscles which assist in the "pumping" of blood; (2) atherosclerosis, a build-up of fatty deposits, including cholesterol, on the inner lining of blood vessels; (3) loss of muscle tone which decreases the effect of body muscle contractions in assisting in the pulsation of blood vessels. Should these circulatory deficiencies occur in the blood vessels supplying the heart muscle with nutrients, the condition is called a coronary heart disease. A heart attack, for example, occurs when a portion of the heart muscle is deprived of blood because of a blood vessel blockage, or clot, in the artery supplying blood to that muscle tissue. The tissue is destroyed, and the heart is made proportionately weaker.

As stated earlier, degeneration is an inevitable process and, given a long enough life span, nearly all people will show clinical signs of degenerative heart disease. This is the primary reason why cardiovascular diseases are by far the leading cause of death in the United States.

That young people are increasingly victimized by degenerative diseases is one of the paradoxes of modern society. Youth and degeneration are contradictory terms. Heart attacks at age 75 and age 45, while causing the same type of tissue damage to the heart muscle, are the results of degeneration produced by different circumstances: one predictable, the other avoidable. Degenerative diseases of youth and middle age are most commonly caused by misuse and abuse of the body and not from normal loss of efficiency which accompanies age.

Misuse and abuse of the body are generally the results of personal and social habits that directly affect the efficiency of the cardiovascular system. Overeating to the point of obesity creates excessive strain on a circulatory system that was designed to "feed" lesser amounts of tissue. Lack of exercise reduces the tone of body muscles and the "pumping" muscles of the heart and circulatory systems. Excessive intake of animal fats may increase cholesterol build-up. Smoking tends to increase the heart rate artificially—that is, when there is no physiological need for the increase—and correspondingly increase blood pressure. All these conditions represent risk factors and will, as shown by the examples in Figures 3.2, increase the likelihood that cardiovascular diseases will occur before their inevitable appearance in old age.

From a medical and community health standpoint, it seems necessary that a greater distinction be made between the preventable forms of cardiovascular disease and the inevitable ones. When health efforts are being employed in both areas, the separation of the two categories is not being clearly made in terms of research money spent, technology employed, social and health services offered, and facilities available. The increasing number of elderly in the population will eventually force the question of priorities be-

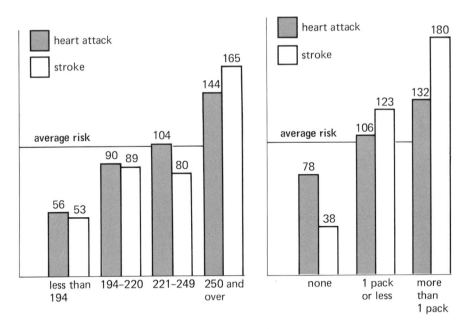

FIGURE 3.2. Personal habits, such as smoking or overconsumption of saturated fats, can increase the risk of cardiovascular disease. *Left:* The relationship between the level of cholesterol in the blood and the risk of heart attack and stroke in men. *Right:* The relationship between cigarette smoking and the risk of heart attack and stroke in men. *(Courtesy of the American Heart Association)*

tween the prolongation of life of the aged and the increased productivity of younger people—a quantity versus quality dilemma. It seems likely that in the near future we will have to make choices between provisions for the young and those for the aged. In fact, the move seems to be well underway, as witnessed by the increasing number of cases of euthanasia, of older people who are voluntarily choosing death over a helpless existence, and of the believers in the new "death ethic" who are promoting an end to life with dignity and respect.

Arthritis. Arthritis is a group of diseases characterized by deterioration and a degree of immobility of the joints of the body. Rheumatoid arthritis and osteoarthritis are the most common types, accounting for 10 million cases of the disease in this country. Death from the disease is infrequent, but discomfort and disability are more common than for any other chronic disorder.

Rheumatoid arthritis produces inflammation and swelling of the joints, characterized by periods of severe pain and immobility. For unknown reasons, it is about three times more common among women than men. Treatment usually includes special exercises, diathermy, rest, and a balanced diet. Permanent crippling is commonly avoided if treatment procedures are routinely followed.

Osteoarthritis is characterized by a softening of the bone ends at the joints. It is a progressively degenerative condition, believed to be the result of aging. Suggested contributing factors are obesity, hard joint usage over a period of time, and a genetic predisposition. Hydrotherapy is the most common treatment, although steroids and hormones are recommended by some specialists.

Like cancer patients, arthritis victims are the target of a large number of unscrupulous "medical" practitioners and manufacturers of pseudo-medical gadgets and nostrums. The progressive degeneration, immobility, and intense pain, coupled with often ineffective medications, produces a desperation that makes "quick relief" products difficult to resist. It is estimated by the Arthritis Foundation that arthritis patients are bilked out of approximately 80 million dollars a year by phoney products with false and misleading claims.

Cancer

Cancer comprises many diseases, each of which has in common the characteristic of abnormal cell growth. The differentiation between these diseases is primarily a matter of location within body tissues—from the bone marrow in leukemia to lung tissue in lung cancer—although there is growing evidence to indicate some distinction among types of cancer according to cause. Nevertheless, cancer is not considered a single disease with common cause, prevention, and treatment. This fact represents perhaps the greatest frustration in medical and research attempts to control cancer, for a great deal of time and effort has been spent in nearly fruitless searches for commonalities of cause and treatment. As will be discussed later, the one common element that may prove the most significant is the body's natural defenses against tumorous growths and/or their causes.

Cancer is currently the second leading cause of death in the United States, striking about one in four persons. Statistically, it is a sporadic disease in the sense that its occurrence varies widely according to age and sex. The age groups with the highest incidence rates of cancer are the 5 to 14 and the 50 to 59 year-old brackets. Thus, the common belief that cancer is a disease of the aged can be laid to rest. The death rate from cancer reflects a highly variable pattern for the years 1930–1975. Male deaths have increased steadily in both white and nonwhite populations, with nonwhite deaths showing a dramatic increase over this period. From 1935 white female deaths have decreased steadily, while nonwhite females show a pattern of increase until 1950 and a steady decrease since then. Trends in mortality rates for males and females are shown in Table 3.1, while comparable incidence percentages are shown in Figure 3.3.

As has been discussed in relationship to many of today's health problems, social and personal factors appear to exert some influence in cancer etiology and treatment. The relationship of smoking to lung cancer has already been discussed in this context. In cancer of genital origin, marital status appears to bear a causal relationship. Cancers of the cervix and prostate occur at a higher rate among married than single persons. A higher incidence of breast cancer has been observed among single women. Early marriage has been related to cancer of the cervix but has also been associated with a lower incidence of breast cancer. Placing these associations in context with suspected causative agents such as viruses, radiation, pollution, and certain environmental and industrial chemicals presents an epidemiological puzzle so complicated as to defy solution, despite the allocation of great amounts of research time and money. Progress is measured in small doses and at great expense.

A further personal-social factor complicates the diagnosis, treatment, and community health approach to cancer. Over the years, the disease has developed emotional overtones to such a degree that some of the population fears the disease and its treatment

TABLE 3.1 Trends in age-adjusted cancer death rates per 100,000 population, 1952–54 to 1967–69*

Sex	Site	1952–54	1967–69	Percent changes	Comments
Male	All Sites	136.0	155.1	+ 14	Steady increase mainly due to lung cancer.
Female	All Sites	118.5	109.6	− 8	Slight decrease.
Male	Breast	0.2	0.2	—	Constant rate.
Female	Breast	21.8	22.9	+ 5	Slight fluctuations: Overall no change.
Male	Colon & Rectum	19.3	18.8	− 3	Slight decrease in both sexes.
Female	Colon & Rectum	18.0	15.8	− 12	
Male	Lung	22.7	44.5	+ 96	Steady increase in both sexes due to cigarette smoking
Female	Lung	4.0	8.1	+103	
Male	Oral	4.6	4.9	+ 7	Slight fluctuations: Overall no change in both sexes.
Female	Oral	1.4	1.4	—	
Male	Skin	2.4	2.5	+ 4	Slight fluctuations: Overall no change in both sexes.
Female	Skin	1.5	1.5	—	
Female	Uterus	17.2	10.6	− 38	Steady decrease attributed in part to widening acceptance of regular checkup with "Pap Test."
Male	Esophagus	3.8	4.1	+ 8	Slight fluctuations: Overall no change in both sexes.
Female	Esophagus	1.1	1.1	—	
Male	Stomach	16.9	9.1	− 46	Steady decrease in both sexes: Reasons unknown.
Female	Stomach	8.7	4.5	− 48	
Male	Pancreas	6.9	8.8	+ 28	Steady increase in both sexes: Reasons unknown.
Female	Pancreas	4.3	5.2	+ 21	
Male	Prostate	14.0	13.5	− 4	Early increase, later decrease, again increasing.
Female	Ovary	7.2	7.6	+ 6	Steady increase.
Male	Kidney	2.9	3.5	+ 21	Steady slight increase.
Female	Kidney	1.7	1.7	—	Slight fluctuations: Overall no change.
Male	Leukemia	6.8	7.3	+ 7	Early increase, later leveling off.
Female	Leukemia	4.7	4.6	− 2	Slight early increase, later leveling off.

* From '73 *Cancer Facts and Figures*, American Cancer Society.

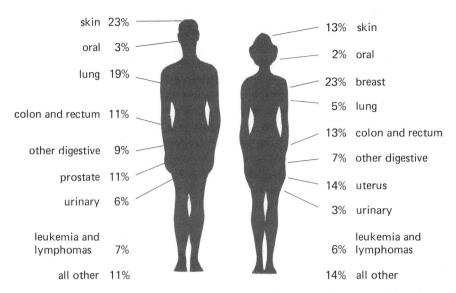

skin 23%

oral 3%

lung 19%

colon and rectum 11%

other digestive 9%

prostate 11%

urinary 6%

leukemia and lymphomas 7%

all other 11%

13% skin

2% oral

23% breast

5% lung

13% colon and rectum

7% other digestive

14% uterus

3% urinary

leukemia and lymphomas 6%

14% all other

FIGURE 3.3.   The percentages of cancer incidence by site and sex. *(Courtesy of the American Cancer Society)*

with an intensity approaching a phobia. Surgery, radiation, and potent chemical treatments are viewed by many as equally dangerous as the disease iself, a view encouraged and promoted by fraudulent medical practitioners, or quacks, who prey on the ignorance and fear of those emotionally unable to accept the realities of cancer. A "painless" or "surgery-free cure" becomes an acceptable though ineffective compromise between fear and a rational approach to the problem.

The coexistence of emotionalism and quackery pose very real and difficult problems to the community health worker, for these factors seriously interfere with attempts to motivate the public to effective action in cancer prevention and treatment. In the face of potent fear, the lure of a "guaranteed, painless relief from cancer without drugs or surgery" can quickly wipe out months of campaigning for early detection, cancer examinations, and surgical-chemical treatments for cancer. This problem is particularly difficult since there are no guarantees that even the best medical technology and treatments will diagnose and cure most types of cancer.

For many years medical research has concentrated its efforts on discovering causes and cures for cancer. Currently, however, a considerable amount of research is being conducted into another aspect of the disease—why is it that three out of four people *do not* get cancer? And why is it that in some instances diagnosed cases of cancer will suddenly show a permanent remission of symptoms? Scientists have produced limited laboratory evidence to suggest that some people possess chemical protection against cancerous growths, a physiological phenomenon not unlike the antigen-antibody reaction that occurs when foreign elements enter the body. The implications of this research are enormous, for it suggests the possibility of developing a means by which all people can receive, by natural or artificial means, a form of chemical immunity against cancer. Perhaps there is after all a commonality that will provide a single method for the effective control of this disease.

Diabetes

Although chronic in nature, diabetes is classified as a constitutional disease, one in which a body part malfunctions because of an apparent structural defect. The pancreas malfunctions in diabetes by the inadequate production of the hormone, insulin. Oxidation of sugar is greatly reduced, resulting in a high blood-sugar level, upsetting other metabolic balances, and leading to diabetic coma. Long-term complications include cardiovascular disease, neuritis, and cataracts.

The precise cause of diabetes is unknown, although genetic factors and obesity have been identified as contributing factors. Over 50 percent of diabetics have a family history of the disease, and it has been estimated that about half of diabetic patients have at one time been 20 percent or more overweight. Age-specific rates reveal a fairly consistent pattern with few cases under 21 years of age, an increasing frequency between 21 and 45, and over 50 percent of the cases developing between the ages of 45 and 60. The estimated total number of cases in this country is about 3 million, and the mortality rate from the disease makes diabetes the sixth leading cause of death in the United States.

From a control standpoint, the important characteristic of diabetes is its insidious nature. It develops slowly and with varying degrees of intensity. Many people are not aware that they have the disease until it has progressed to the point where control is difficult. Detected in its early stages, diabetes can often by controlled by dietary means without insulin supplementation. In addition, the mortality rate from cases diagnosed early is one-third that of those diagnosed after severe complications have occurred.

Mass attempts at diabetes control, therefore, have been directed at early diagnosis, implementing screening programs using urine and blood samples, and concentrating on families with genetic histories of diabetes, persons who are overweight, and persons over 40 years of age. Recently, mass screening programs in the communities, available to anyone, have been heavily promoted and sponsored by various official and voluntary groups.

Chronic Obstructive Lung Diseases

To the health and medical profession, the recent increases in the incidence of chronic lung diseases caused by inspiration of foreign substances have been alarming. The decrease in lung diseases of a pathogenic nature, such as pneumonia and tuberculosis, since 1950 has to an extent been counteracted by a corresponding increase

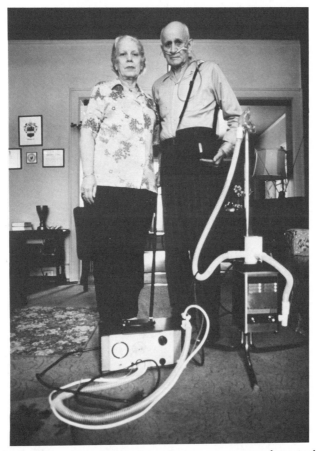

Before his death, this man was totally dependent on pure oxygen from equipment carried wherever he went. He was suffering from emphysema after working 50 years with the railroad and living in Birmingham, Alabama, one of the severely air-polluted urban areas in the United States. *(EPA-DOCUMERICA, LeRoy Woodson)*

in diseases such as chronic bronchitis, emphysema, chronic asthma, and lung cancer. There is some justification to the argument that the increase is a function of the larger elderly population since the obstructive lung diseases hit hardest at persons over 50 years of age. However, there is sufficient evidence to indicate that certain environmental and social factors, such as air pollution and smoking, contribute to the increase.

Because the concern over the chronic obstructive lung diseases has arisen only recently, health and medical programs are still in the pioneering stages. The National Tuberculosis Association, now the National Lung Association, has assumed leadership in the community health aspects of screening and detection. The emergence of national concern over smoking, air pollution, and black lung disease among coal miners has led to some federal involvement in diagnostic and rehabilitative programs. In view of the severity of these problems, there seems little doubt that additional efforts from voluntary and official agencies will soon be forthcoming.

NUTRITIONAL PROBLEMS

While other health problems, such as pollution and drug abuse, have been receiving the greatest amount of "press" in the United States, a great deal of concern about nutritional problems has been recently generated. Studies conducted in 1950 and early 1960 described patterns of malnutrition and dietary deficiencies, but were ignored because they were felt to have been derived from "faulty and imprecise data-gathering techniques." In 1968, a group called The Citizen's Board of Inquiry Into Hunger and Malnutrition presented a devastating testimony of hunger and malnutrition in the land of plenty. It estimated that 10 million Americans are underfed or malnourished. About that same time, CBS television presented a special documentary, "Hunger in America," with evidence supportive of The Citizen's Board report—an event that brought the problem visually and dramatically to millions of homes in America. Bits and pieces of evidence then began to accumulate: a diagnosed case of rickets in New York City; cases of starvation in Indian settlements and isolated Appalachian communities; and children blinded because of Vitamin A deficiencies. Concerned nutritionists, physicians, and health workers began to view with great alarm the hard evidence of serious nutritional deficiencies among the best-fed people in the world.

The most complete assessment of the nutritional status of the United States population was initiated by the Department of Health,

Education, and Welfare. Preliminary reports from the National Nutrition Survey began to appear in early 1970. The study centered on randomly selected populations in ten states, with emphasis on poverty-level families. The evidence presents a profile of nutritional inadequacies that would be considered disgraceful in many less wealthy nations.

While the findings of many studies apply mainly to poverty-level populations, the inference should not be drawn that this group is unique in its nutritional problems. Although accurate figures are not available for the general population, studies of nutritional status agree that there are widespread dietary deficiencies in both sexes and across all age levels. At other than poverty levels, the problems are related mainly to dietary selection rather than food supply—eating the right foods as opposed to having enough food to eat. Such nutritional problems may result from (1) failure to ingest food because of anorexia, restrictive cultural taboos, or serious dental problems; (2) failure to utilize food because of metabolic diseases or intestinal infections that prevent assimilation or absorption of nutrients; or (3) failure to fulfill increased nutritional requirements produced by childhood and adolescence, pregnancy and lactation, heavy physical labor, and other circumstances that increase metabolism.

Obesity has been indicated as the most widespread form of mal-

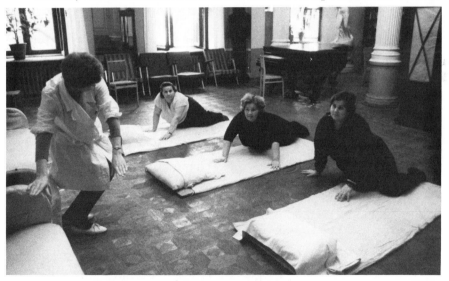

Malnutrition is by no means restricted to poor and underdeveloped nations; it is common in many of the most affluent societies. Above, a nutritional clinic helps obese individuals cope with their problem through physical exercise and special diets. *(Courtesy of the World Health Organization)*

nutrition in this country today. Estimates of people who are overweight (10 percent above ideal weight) run as high as 45 percent of the population, while obesity (20 percent or more above ideal weight) is said to be a problem with about 30 percent of the population. Incidence of obesity increases with age after early adulthood and is higher in women than men after age 30.

Obesity in children is a particularly difficult problem. Recent evidence indicates that obese children run a high risk of becoming obese adults. It is estimated for a child obese at age 12, the odds against attaining normal weight in adulthood are 4 to 1, and if the problem exists at the end of adolescence, the odds increase to 28 to 1. Unfortunately, the notion that chubbiness equals good health in children is still widespread.

The etiology of obesity involves a complex of factors—physical, emotional, and cultural—but is unfortunately viewed by many, particularly the slim, as little more than lack of self-discipline. Obese and overweight individuals are easy targets for the promoters of various reducing programs and products which often produce a cycle of physical and mental ups and downs that is often more dangerous than the obesity itself.

The problem of obesity is further compounded by the societal idealization of slimness. Being even the slightest bit overweight is often viewed as a serious problem, especially among young adults who often measure the severity of a weight problem in terms of aesthetics rather than health. Deficient diets, inadequate eating patterns, fatigue, and a host of disease susceptibilities are not unusual consequences from attempts to control weight in accordance with social, rather than medical, standards.

The needs of our society in relation to nutritional problems are many. We need first of all a distribution system that provides an adequate supply of proper nutrients to all people in this country. The right to health certainly includes access to the most basic of all man's needs. Secondly, we need the kind of sound nutrition education that pays heed not only to purchasing and cooking, but to the multitude of personal and social factors that exert such strong influence on eating habits. Thirdly, we need extensive research in all areas related to food consumption and nutritional status. Information is far from complete on nutritional subjects ranging from the value of food additives to motivational stimuli in eating to the full extent of malnutrition. Finally, we need to extend our health services and programs beyond piecemeal provision of food to the poor to public, noncommercial sources of assistance in weight control, examinations to determine dietary deficiencies, counseling services, and so forth. The relationship of poor nutrition to a host of disease conditions warrants more organized community health involvement in the prevention and amelioration of this increasingly serious health problem.

TOPICS FOR DISCUSSION

1. Discuss the reasons for the substantial and potentially dangerous increase in the use of antibiotics from the standpoints of (1) the doctor and (2) the health consumer. Identify some ways the community health profession might work to relieve this problem.
2. Discuss the differences between inevitable and preventable cardiovascular diseases. If you had the sole authority to dispense all money available for research, prevention, and treatment of cardiovascular diseases, how would you distribute the money between the inevitable and preventable cardiovascular disease programs? Be prepared to defend your answer.

4. Man's Social and Environmental Health

MENTAL ILLNESSES

It was but a few decades ago that the medical profession accepted the arbitrary division of people into two categories of mental status: sane and insane, or normal and abnormal. Such distinctions, of course, have been discarded as inaccurate and potentially damaging, and it is now recognized that a continuous spectrum of behavior exists between the well-adjusted personality and clinically-diagnosed psychotic behavior. This spectrum is similar to that of physical illnesses, ranging from optimum physical well-being to definite illness.

The problem of definition for mental illness is much more difficult than for physical illnesses because of the wide range of acceptable behavior in our society and the absence of definitive diagnostic tools. Outward behavior is the only real measure of an individual's state of mental health, and, since the human mind has an infinite capacity to direct and redirect behavior at any given point in time, such behavior is at best unreliable as a clinical source of measurement for diagnosing and classifying mental illnesses.

Obvious and prolonged deviations from normal and realistic behavior, however, are not difficult for the trained professional to diagnose as a severe, psychotic mental illness. To identify the cause of a given illness and prescribe definitive treatment based on the cause is a more difficult task. The first diagnostic problem is to determine if the cause is in fact psychological, for a large number of mental illnesses are of organic, or physiological, origin. Brain-tissue damage which may produce behavioral symptoms of a psychotic nature can be caused by a number of factors: an interrupted blood flow to the brain, as in senility, strokes, or brain tumors; the presence of infectious organisms, such as the spirochete in advanced syphilis; or prolonged exposure to chemicals, such as heroin or alcohol.

If a psychotic patient is found to be free of such organic causes, then by the process of elimination the cause is classified as psychological in nature. However unsophisticated this may appear, it reflects the extent to which behavioral problems have thus far eluded distinct and accurate classifications by cause. Recent physiological research has suggested the strong possibility that deviant behavior, particularly of an aggressive nature, may in some instances be due to abnormal genetic structure. Similar research indicates that some forms of psychotic behavior may have a biochemical base. Research on LSD and other hallucinogens has established the fact that minute amounts of chemical substances can produce profound personality changes. The possibility of similar aberrations resulting from involuntary changes in the complicated structure of the brain is the subject of intensive biochemical research. As definitive research discoveries are made, the process of diagnosing and treating mental illnesses by cause will reach a more scientific and productive level.

While severe psychotic illnesses are in most cases readily observable, lesser forms of mental and emotional disturbances are more difficult to detect and diagnose. The old saying that "everyone's odd but me and thee and sometimes I wonder about thee" is very much to the point. All people exhibit degrees of deviant behavior at times and with varying degrees of intensity. The point at which such behavior becomes an illness worthy of treatment is indistinct at best. The key elements in such a determination are usually identified as the length of duration and the intensity of the symptoms, be they depression, fear, anxiety, aggression, and so forth. When such emotional or mental symptoms persist or are severe to the point where one's normal life style is greatly altered or relationships with others seriously deteriorating, then the behavior reaches the point of illness and indicates treatment is needed. Although many people continue to reject treatment even under these circumstances, those who do seek it have, by their actions, defined their condition as an illness and are seeking release from the behavioral symptoms. Thus, statistical descriptions of the extent of mental illnesses in this country will normally include those who have diagnosable psychotic disturbances and those who seek, or are forced by their actions, to receive treatment for a variety of disturbances that are interfering with their normal and acceptable patterns of behavior.

There are a number of criteria used in determining the relative

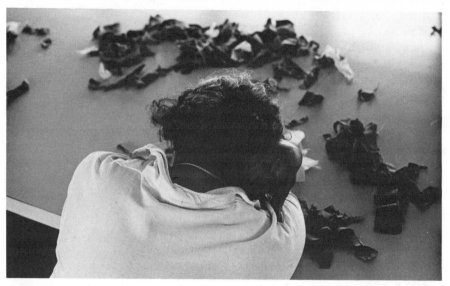

Mental illnesses cannot as yet be scientifically classified; the causes of symptomatic behavior can range from chemical or neurological imbalances in the body to an inability to cope with the stresses of modern society. More often than not, the individual himself, rather than a clinical specialist, must be the first to define his condition as illness by seeking treatment for it. For this reason, many cases go undiagnosed and untreated. *(Courtesy of the World Health Organization)*

severity of health problems: death rate, morbidity rates, economic impact, and so forth. However, if a health problem is evaluated in terms of the extent to which it results in loss of human productivity and societal contributions, mental illnesses would have to be the number-one health problem in this country. No other single group of illnesses produces such long-term debility in so many people. As far back as 1963, President Kennedy stated his concern over the severity of this problem: "They (mental illnesses) occur more frequently, affect more people, require more prolonged treatment, cause more suffering by the families of the afflicted, waste more of our human resources, and constitute more financial drain upon both the public treasury and the personal finances of the individual families than any other single condition."

The statistical description of the extent of mental disturbances as presented below is persuasive evidence of the degree to which this condition decreases the human resources of this country.

1. On any given day, there are approximately 770,000 persons who are hospitalized for mental illnesses. This is a number greater than the combined total of all other patients hospitalized for any other reason.

2. An estimated 20 million Americans are in need of treatment for mental disturbances. Of that number, about 3 million are actually receiving needed treatment.

3. One out of every 10 children born each year will need hospitalized treatment of mental illnesses at some time during his or her life. Approximately 15 years ago the estimation was 1 in 12.

4. Approximately half of those admitted to mental institutions have had at least one previous admission.

5. An estimated 2.5 billion dollars are spent each year for state and private treatment of mental illnesses. The economic burden is dramatically increased by an estimated loss of 7 billion dollars per year in consumer purchasing power and productivity in industry.

6. The vast majority of mental patients are housed in state hospitals which provide approximately 500,000 beds. More than 75 percent of these hospitals were built during the early 1900s, and some have been condemned as hazardous.

7. The average physician-to-patient ratio is about 1:100 with some larger hospitals having a much higher ratio.

8. Approximately 18 dollars per patient is the average daily expenditure for maintenance. This compares to approximately 100 dollars in other types of hospitals. However minimal the amount, the burden on state treasuries is great and represents a tempting item for budget cuts.

9. New admissions to mental hospitals have about a 70 percent chance of being released within a year. After two years, the chances are about 1 in 16, and after 5 years, the odds skyrocket to 99 to 1.

10. It is estimated that more than 10 percent of America's school children are emotionally disturbed, and some as early as kindergarten have diagnosable psychotic conditions.

As startling as these statistics are, they obviously do not tell the whole story. Because of the insidious nature of the diseases and their social implications, many people will not seek treatment for emotional problems and others will not admit their existence. Thus, the "hidden" incidence of these illnesses is not reflected in the statistics. In addition, not all psychogenic diseases are included in the statistical description. Large numbers of patients are being treated by physicians for physical ailments, of which all or some factors in their etiology are psychological. One estimate runs as high as one in every two patients. Three of the five leading causes of death among the 15–25 age group are to a degree psychogenic in origin —accidents, suicide, and murder.

Although it can be argued that the statistical picture of mental illness is somewhat inflated because of better diagnostic procedures and an increased willingness of people to seek care, the evidence strongly indicates a trend toward a substantial increase in the number of emotionally disturbed children and adults. If standards used to evaluate the score of infectious diseases were applied to mental illnesses, the problem could be legitimately termed an "epidemic out of control."

Such a term would indicate that the medical and psychiatric capacities are not keeping pace with the increase in the number of emotionally disturbed children and adults. However true this may be, the fact remains that a major revolution in the treatment and rehabilitation of the mentally ill has been taking place over the past two decades. The discovery and application in the 1950s of tranquilizing and antidepressant drugs made it possible to control the symptoms of some mental patients, allowing longer periods of stability and increased communication and providing a more suitable environment for psychotherapeutic treatment. Using drug therapy, many patients are able to leave the closed community of the mental hospital and return to the outside world. While periodically receiving out-patient treatment, the patient can live at home, hold down a job, and be a contributing member of society.

The rapid return of patients from mental institutions to the community and the recognition that prevention is the best method of control created an urgent need to increase the capacity of local communities to provide psychiatric facilities and personnel. In the early 1960s some states passed legislation creating regional and community psychiatric facilities and authorizing the closure or reorganization of state mental institutions. In 1963 Congress passed the Community Mental Health Centers Act, authorizing Federal support and financing of direct mental health services. On a matching fund basis, nearly 500 localities in the United States have established mental health centers and auxiliary services such as hot lines and crisis intervention centers.

The decentralization of mental health services from state to local jurisdiction is significant in several ways. It is in keeping with the general trend toward consumer participation in health programming and with the philosophy that local control leads to more active utilization and support by local citizens. Efforts by communities to establish such centers are also an indication that the community recognizes and accepts mental disturbances as treatable illnesses—an attitude of acceptance that provides the patient with the

comfort of knowing that his treatment will not be socially stigma-
tized. Perhaps of greatest importance, community health centers
provide for the first time a convenient avenue of assistance for the
"average" citizen who suffers from the "average" crises of daily
living—the death of a loved one, the pressures of a job, the problems
of adolescence. Never before have organized programs been available to the great majority of people who on occasion need supportive
psychotherapy by trained professionals. This kind of intervention
is the best form of prevention.

The transition in practice and attitude from long-term care to
outpatient treatment is at present in its early stages. Resistance to
change is evident in some communities which refuse to consider
local treatment facilities. Political and economic restrictions have
been posed by other communities which have been reluctant to
close state mental institutions in their vicinity. While proceeding in
haste is potentially as harmful as resisting change, it appears most
likely that an accelerated pace of decentralization of mental health
services has the greatest potential for providing a public program
for satisfactory psychiatric care.

Drug Abuse

The current concern over drug abuse in this country is as strong
as for nearly any other health problem in the nation's history. Yet
the abuse of drugs has been a consistent part of our culture with a
history nearly as old as the country itself. For example, the opiates
were potent ingredients in many of the elixirs sold off the back of
covered wagons in traveling medicine shows; heroin was at one
time used for the treatment of narcotics addiction; and the reformed
alcoholic was often kept in a stupor by the administration of an
opium concoction. It is estimated that around the turn of the century
there were nearly 1 million people who were addicted to some form
of opiate.

By comparison, it seems contradictory indeed for the modern
world to exhibit such great concern over an addiction problem that
presently claims only 300,000 victims. The comparison is misleading, however, because abuse in the past was often unintentional and
the addict a victim of ignorance, consuming a medicinal substance
that was legal and acceptable both as a palliative and an elixir.
Abuse by today's addict, on the other hand, is usually deliberate, for
in most instances he is fully aware of the consequences of his actions and that his behavior is both legally and socially unacceptable.
The abuse of a drug today, while often causing strong physical dependence, is often symptomatic of a mental-psychological disorder

in the abuser, and it represents a social as well as medical problem of the highest order.

The extent of the drug problem in this country is unknown. Estimates are grossly inconsistent, mainly because of differing definitions of drug abuse, addiction, and dependence and lack of agreement as to how much is too much and for what purpose. A drug is typically defined as any substance that is used to alter the physical and mental functioning of the body. Drug abuse, therefore, implies the deliberate misuse of a drug. Medicines used for purposes other than medically intended; weight reduction pills used to stay awake or provide energy; doubling a prescribed dosage to get faster action —each represents a common form of drug abuse. It should be noted, however, that "drugs" are often also defined along social and cultural rather than medical lines, with the result that "drug abuse" is often applied only to the consumption of certain drugs and not to the consumption, even in large quantities, of others whose use is considered socially acceptable or even desirable. It is therefore im-

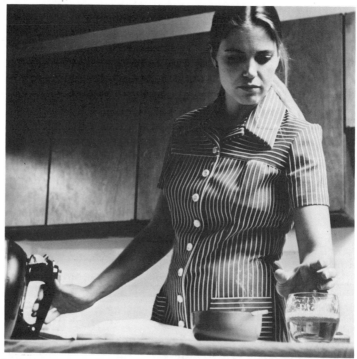

"If you drink while you do the ironing, send the ironing out" reads the caption to one of the many posters put out by the National Institute on Alcohol Abuse and Alcoholism in efforts to educate the public about alcohol and alcoholism in contemporary society. *(NIAAA, Health Services and Mental Health Administration)*

portant to emphasize that the standard to be considered in the determination of instances of drug abuse is not necessarily the one set by public opinion.

According to the more accurate definition of abuse as the misuse of a drug, the most commonly abused drugs are caffeine, nicotine, and alcohol: substances which by a cultural definition would be considered nondrugs. By every conceivable measure—extent of use, number of regular users, amount consumed, money spent, and man-hours under the influence of—the use of these three drugs is greater than that of any of the other psychoactive substances. The medical and social damage done by alcohol and nicotine alone vastly exceeds the physical harm done by all other psychoative drugs put together. In 1970 Americans spent 15.7 billion dollars for alcoholic beverages, 9 billion dollars for tobacco, and 3.2 billion dollars for caffeine beverages—a total of nearly 28 billion dollars! The further expenditure for medical problems directly produced by these substances raises the consumer costs to astronomical levels.

The United States supports a drinking population in excess of 70 million. Of those, approximately 10 percent are classified as having a severe drinking problem. Assuming conservatively that half of this group is married and has at least one child, the resulting toll of lives severely affected by alcoholism is well over 17 million people. The human cost associated with alcohol use is further evidenced by the statistics presented in Table 4.1.

This nation consumes 2.6 gallons of pure alcohol per person; and its consumption generates 10 billion dollars worth of business annually to support one of the largest industries in the country. Additional revenue is generated for governmental treasuries at state and national levels in the form of liquor licenses and taxes. Ironic indeed is the fact that some of this revenue is returned to the drink-

TABLE 4.1   Estimated percentages of destructive events which are related to use of alcohol

Event	Percent related to use of alcohol
Violent death	30
Suicides	25
Fatal highway accidents	54
Pedestrian deaths	30
Prison admissions	30
Accidents other than traffic and industrial	24
Divorces	20

ing public in the form of treatment programs for alcoholics. The sequence of events is a vicious cycle—the more effective the advertising, the greater the drinking population, the larger the profits of the industry, the more substantial the amount of money available (theoretically) for the treatment of problem drinkers. If, as research suggests, alcoholic parents are more likely to have alcoholic children, the spiraling cycle is complete.

In the face of our extensive problem with drug abuse, the most pressing need at the moment is to create a national sense of perspective that places all drugs in the "dangerous" category and all acts of misuse, accidental or intentional, as evidence of a potential health problem. While overreactive prohibitions would cause more problems than they would cure, basic acceptance of the danger inherent in all drugs is a logical and necessary point of departure for effective planning and abuse control programs. Inconsistencies that produce punishment for the use of some drugs and encouragement

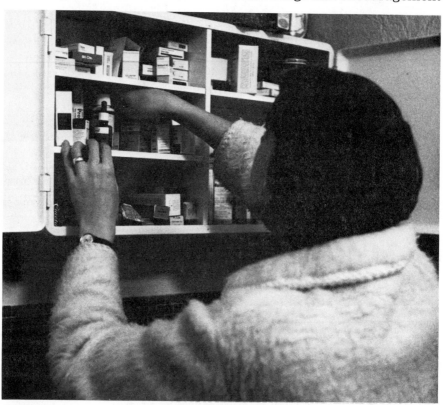

The abuse of drugs is not restricted to those gotten illegally. Many of today's misused and overused drugs can be found in the family medicine chest. *(Courtesy of the World Health Organization)*

for the use of more costly and dangerous ones reflect an hyprocrisy that many people so soundly decry. Pills for going to sleep, staying awake, losing weight, gaining weight, preventing constipation, curing hemorrhoids, and so on, clog the family medicine chest. With no more than the price of purchase, the consumer has available 76 different dandruff shampoos, 48 ointments for boils, 287 remedies for athlete's foot, 14 applications for chapped lips, no less, than 325 analgesics for soothing muscular aches, and an untold number of combination drugs for the relief of pain. How many "users" are the first to condemn their child's experimentation with the more "dangerous" and illicit drugs? There seems little doubt that a large number of addicts and dependent users could trace their habits back to their family medicine cabinets.

TRAUMATIC ILLNESSES

Traumatic illnesses are here defined as bodily injuries resulting from contact with external agents. Such contact may be of a violent nature, such as automobile accidents, occupational injuries, or fires, or of a more insidious nature, as with chemical pollutants or radiation particles. While traumatic illnesses are expected to occur in all societies, the nature and extent of such occurrences are determined by the technology and cultural values of given societies. Injuries resulting from tribal aggressions and hunting accidents may be relatively high in primitive societies, but those resulting from technological pollutions and automobile accidents do not constitute serious threats to health in those societies.

There is danger, however, with the temptation to generalize about progress and technology and in the very simplicity by which traumatic illnesses are defined and identified. The tendency is to define and identify them in purely physical terms, and such a tendency belies the tremendous complexity of the problem. Beyond merely the physical nature of traumatic diseases are the biological, ecological, and economic factors which in combination magnify the scope of the problem beyond the mere prevention of accidents, "cleaning up" the air, and eliminating all industrial uses of radiation. That severe health problems result from these environmental conditions is a foregone conclusion; that these problems exist within the context of a highly complex industrial and social structure based in large measure on the very elements that produce the environmental conditions is a severe obstacle to prevention and control of traumatic illnesses.

The discussion of all the economic, political, and ecological ramifications of traumatic disease control is beyond the scope of this book. As with other health problems, the community health worker is well advised to consider the broader context within which traumatic illnesses occur, for without such consideration, preventive programs will produce only meager results.

Accidents

Accidents resulting from sudden, unexpected impact with environmental objects or exposure to poisonous chemicals are the fourth leading cause of fatalities in the United States, a position which has remained unchanged since 1948 (see Table 4.2). The scope of this problem becomes even greater, however, when the total loss due to accidents is considered. The number of deaths from accidents has increased steadily since 1903, with 117,000 deaths occurring in 1973. Even though the death rate for accidents has decreased steadily due to population growth, the rate of accidental death in ages 1 to 44 is higher than any other single cause of death (see Table 4.3). More children from ages 1 to 14 die from accidents than from the next six leading causes combined; in the age group 15 to 24, accidents cause more deaths than all other causes put together. As shown on Table 4.4, over 11 million disabling injuries from accidents occurred in 1973, resulting in well over twice that many man-days of work lost and 30 billion dollars in medical expenses, property damages and insurance claims. The total cost of human suffering and permanent incapacitation is, of course, incalculable.

Accidents are generally classified according to the place in which they occur: in motor vehicles, at work, at home, and in public places. As seen in Table 4.4, over half of all accidental deaths occur

TABLE 4.2   Accidental deaths and death rates, United States*

Year	Number of deaths (average)	Deaths per 100,000 population (average)	Rank as cause of death
1933–1942	98,765	76.2	5
1943–1947	97,561	71.4	5
1948–1952	93,280	61.8	4
1953–1957	93,719	57.1	4
1958–1962	97,176	51.9	4
1963–1966	113,000	57.7	4
1967–1971	114,000	56.8	4
1971–1973	117,000	55.9	4

* From the National Center for Health Statistics

in motor vehicles, including those deaths which occur in industrial and agricultural settings. Although the death rate from motor vehicle accidents has declined in terms of population growth and number of miles driven, they still rank as the leading cause of death in ages 1 to 24, and the third leading cause in ages 25 to 44. Conspicuous

TABLE 4.3   Leading causes of death by age, United States, 1970*

Age group and cause of death	Number of deaths	Death rates per 100,000
1 to 4 Years	11,548	85
Accidents	4,300	32
Motor-vehicle	1,572	12
Drowning	800	6
Fires, burns	713	5
Falls	205	2
Ingestion of food, object	201	1
Other	809	6
Congenital anomalies	1,331	10
Cancer	1,027	8
5 to 14 Years	16,847	41
Accidents	8,203	20
Motor-vehicle	4,159	10
Drowning	1,550	4
Fires, burns	609	1
Other	1,885	5
Cancer	2,429	6
Congenital anomalies	901	2
15 to 24 Years	45,261	127
Accidents	24,336	68
Motor-vehicle	16,720	47
Drowning	2,330	7
Poison (solid, liquid)	1,010	3
Firearms	726	2
Other	3,550	9
Homicide	4,157	12
Suicide	3,128	9
25 to 44 Years	111,810	232
Accidents	23,979	50
Motor-vehicle	13,446	28
Drowning	1,520	3
Falls	1,111	2
Fires, burns	1,003	2
Other	6.899	15
Heart disease	18,238	38
Cancer	17,841	37

* From the National Safety Council, *Accident Facts* 1974 Edition

increases in pedestrian deaths and bicycle and motorcycle fatalities have been noted in the past decade.

The home is the setting for approximately one-fourth of all accidental deaths, with the very young and the very old the most frequent victims. Falls account for over 50 percent of all such fatalities. Fires and gas inhalation have become increasingly common causes of death, as have accidents involving firearms, 50 percent of which occur in the home. Similar factors, with the addition of drownings, are the most common causes of accidental deaths in public places such as recreational areas, municipal buildings, and public parks.

Places of work are potentially the most hazardous of all accident sites because of the constant exposure of workers to high-speed machinery and industrial chemicals. Yet the death rate in occupational settings is the lowest of all sites, and fewer disabling injuries occur at work than at home or in public places. Accident prevention programs, spurred by workman compensation laws, are stringently enforced in American industry and consistently monitored to maintain safety equipment and encourage safe working conditions. The Occupational Safety and Health Act was enacted in 1970 to provide safety inspection and accident reporting systems in order to build even more systemized monitoring procedures. Community and safety specialists would do well to study the methods and techniques by which successful occupational safety programs have been imple-

TABLE 4.4 Principal classes of accident, United States, 1973*

Class	Deaths	Change from 1972	Disabling injuries
Motor Vehicle	55,800	−1%	2,000,000
Public nonwork	51,800		1,900,000
Work	3,800		100,000
Home	200		10,000
Work	14,200	+1%	2,500,000
Nonmotor vehicle	10,400		2,400,000
Motor vehicle	3,800		100,000
Home	26,000	−4%	4,100,000
Nonmotor vehicle	25,800		4,100,000
Motor vehicle	200		10,000
Public†	25,000	+6%	3,000,000

* From the National Safety Council, *Accident Facts,* 1974 Edition
† Excludes motor-vehicle and work accidents in public places. Includes recreation (swimming, hunting, etc.), transportation except motor vehicle, public building accidents, etc.

mented. The adaptation of these procedures to other health and safety programs may prove valuable.

While accidents appear on the surface to be more controllable and preventable than other contemporary health problems, in reality the problem is much the same in terms of complexity and elusiveness. Despite the relative effectiveness of safety programs in teaching the skills of safe behavior and the development of safer automobiles and equipment, the number of accidents and deaths continues to increase. As with other contemporary health problems, the dominant causative factors in accidents are social and behavioral. Ninety-three percent of all automobile accidents are due to "improper driving" where human error, rather than lack of driving

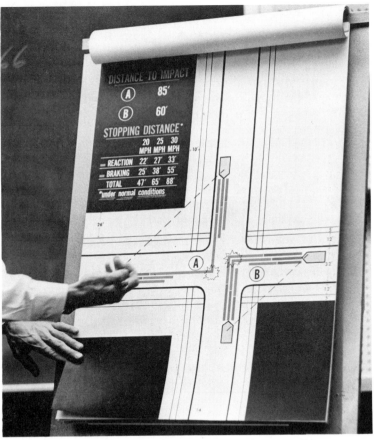

The National Safety Council sponsors many community and correspondence courses on automobile safety; the above is part of its defensive driver course. It is believed, however, that the majority of automobile accidents result, not from ignorance or lack of skill on the driver's part, but rather from social or behavioral factors, such as intoxication or dare-devil driving. (Courtesy of the National Safety Council)

skills, was the cause. Over one-half of all fatal accidents involved at least one driver who was under the influence of alcohol. An unknown number of suicides, either by an overdose of pills or single-car fatalities, are classified as accidents. Seat belts are not worn an estimated 60 percent of the time for personal reasons, resulting in an estimated 7,500 deaths per year. When classified in social and behavioral terms, the causative factors in accidents are not unlike those of mental illnesses, drug abuse, heart diseases, and so forth.

A factor which further complicates the problem of accident prevention and control is the very nature of accidents which by definition are unexpected and unavoidable occurrences. A certain number of accidents are going to happen regardless of efforts to prevent them, particularly efforts related to teaching safety skills and providing a safe environment. There exists a point at which accidents cannot be prevented—an irreducible minimum. While identifying that point may be difficult, little effort has been devoted to doing so, and in the meantime increasing amounts of money continue to be spent in attempts to further refine already successful accident prevention programs. In addition, a great deal more effort should be devoted to identifying the human factors responsible for accidents and to incorporating such behaviorally oriented material into existing safety education programs.

Environmental Pollution

Not even the most casual observer of the public media of recent months and years could be unaware of the chorus of warning and doom emanating from qualified scientists, conservationists, and politicians concerning the technological destruction of our environment. In the name of progress, new and advanced technology provides more convenience, efficiency, and speed to our lives while progressively depleting the exhaustible supply of natural resources and living space. Man's dominion over nature, his desire to streamline and chromeplate his surroundings, to manipulate time and space to his convenience, and yet his persistent desire to return to the simple life, to the beauty and serenity of nature, presents a paradox of the highest order.

Among the most critical by-products of man's technological progress has been an ever-increasing effluence of destructive chemicals into the air, water, and biological environment. In a normal year, the United States produces 142 million tons of smoke and fumes, 20 million tons of waste paper, 50 trillion gallons of industrial sewage, and an unknown amount of industrial and agricultural

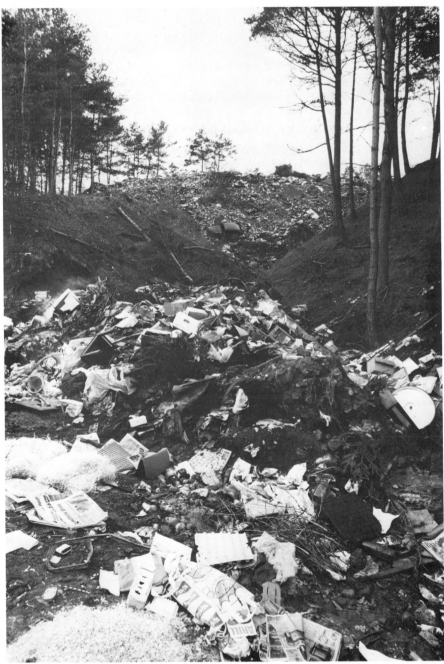

Man's failure to control the growth and by-products of his technology has often resulted in the destruction of nature and natural beauty. *(Courtesy of the World Health Organization)*

biocides. The full extent to which environmental pollution presents a health threat is at present unknown because of the recency of the phenomenon and an inability to predict its long-term effects. Even to the limited extent that the effects of environmental pollution are currently known, however, the threat to health and longevity is indeed a real one.

Air Pollution. Air pollution is generally defined as the presence in the atmosphere of substances in sufficient quantities to be potentially injurious to living things. We have come to include among those substances nearly all elements produced by man and released into the air, some of which are not known to be directly injurious but are suspected to be potentially so. Man-made air pollutants come from industrial and automotive exhausts, home heating, incineration, and crop-spraying.

Most air pollution occurs in two different forms of smog: sulfur

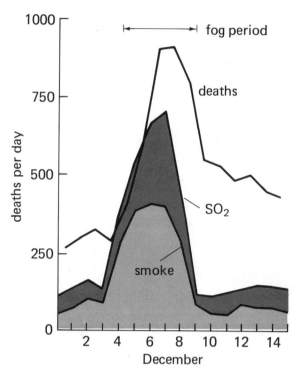

FIGURE 4.1. In December 1952 a "pea-soup" fog settled over London for five days. The subsequent lethal combination of the fog with the already polluted air containing sulfur dioxide and particulate matter from burning coal was implicated in the 4,000 excess deaths recorded during that period. *(From* Committee on Air Pollution, Interim Report. *London: Her Majesty's Stationery Office, December 1953)*

dioxide smog and photochemical smog. Sulfur dioxide smog results from the burning of coal and fuel oil which releases large quantities of sulfur dioxide into the air. Particularly during humid weather, this chemical in combination with other pollutants is absorbed into the sensitive linings of the eye, nose, and respiratory tract, causing irritation and damage. In addition, such pollutants can inhibit ciliary action in the respiratory tract, allowing particulate matter to remain in the lung tissue and cause damage. Chronic bronchitis, bronchial asthma, emphysema, and lung cancer are possible results. While additional research is needed to establish the extent of health problems resulting from sulfur dioxide and combined pollutants, there is substantial empirical evidence to warn communities of the potential hazards. In the first week in December 1930 in the Meuse Valley of Belgium, a highly industrialized area, a heavy air mass held a blanket of smog over the city. Over a thousand residents became ill and 16 died, ten times the normal rate. In October 1948 in Donora, Pennsylvania, 17 deaths were reported under similar conditions, and an additional 42 percent of the population became ill. Also documented are instances in which plant life has been destroyed by sulfur dioxide released from industrial processes such as smelting of silver, copper and zinc. Without proper controls, surrounding vegetation can be completely devastated.

In recent years, the reduction in the use of coal as a fuel and the adoption of procedures to prevent the release of sulfur dioxide have significantly reduced, but not eliminated, this source of air pollution. However, the advent of the internal combustion engine and the prolific use of automobiles led to the emergence of photochemical smog. This type of smog is the combined result of large quantities of internal combustion engine exhaust and weather conditions, specifically frequent periods of sunshine. The energy in sunlight interacts with the pollutants from engine exhaust to produce the type of brownish smog typically present in any major city during sunny weather.

Pollutants in photochemical smog are irritants in themselves and when combined with other pollutants, including sulfur dioxide, produce potentially hazardous conditions. Carbon monoxide is one of the by-products of this interaction. Although concentrations have not reached dangerously high levels generally, high concentrations do occur in heavy traffic periods. In addition, the additive effects of carbon monoxide from cigarette smoking and inhalation from environmental sources may approach a dangerous level. Hydrocarbons, nitrous oxide, and ozone present in photochemical smog are also harmful to plant life and potentially dangerous to man if concentrations increase significantly.

Water Pollution. Water is the most abundant compound on earth and is among the few absolute necessities for the existence of life forms. Its uses have multiplied many times during our present technological era but not without serious and potentially disastrous consequences.

For use internally by man, water is cleansed of microorganisms and high mineral content by simple filtration and chlorination processes. However, the more abundant the elements to be removed, the more difficult the purification process and the more urgent the need to do so. Our present problem with water pollution, simply stated, is that the water is becoming so contaminated with man-made pollutants, that it is not only becoming unusable in its natural state, but is increasingly difficult to purify.

Water becomes polluted from four major sources: sewage, industrial wastes, drainage containing fertilizers and pesticides, and recreational uses of water. Sewage is generally described as waste water generated by home and industry. Sewage treatment facilities are used to "purify" the water of sewage and release it into a local water course. Unfortunately, much of the water containing sewage is inadequately treated or not treated at all in those instances where

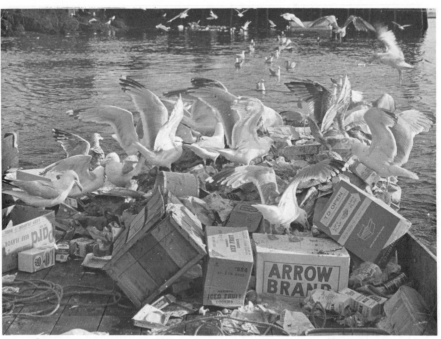

The upsetting of natural ecosystems is one serious result of water pollution. *(Ray Hunold, from National Audubon Society)*

industrial wastes are dumped directly into a lake or stream. Inadequately treated, the sewage can cause chemical and biologic reactions which upset the ecological balance of water courses causing destruction of acquatic life. Lake Erie is the most striking example of this process. The plankton in the lake began to thrive as more and more chemicals were dumped into it. In time, the layer of plankton on the surface of the water had grown so thick that it blocked the sunlight to the lower depths, thus killing many of the fish below.

While the upsetting of biological ecosystems is a potentially devastating process, an equally pressing danger of water pollution is the increasingly difficult process of purifying polluted water for human and industrial uses. Water for these purposes normally comes from surface water such as lakes and streams or from ground sources such as wells or springs. As these sources become more polluted, existing treatment facilities will no longer be adequate for purification purposes. Without proper treatment, waste then becomes a hazardous, disease-producing substance in the sense that infectious microorganisms or poisonous chemicals such as insecticides may survive the treatment process. Some communities at present are faced with the necessity of installing very expensive water-treatment facilities or face the real hazards of a polluted community water supply.

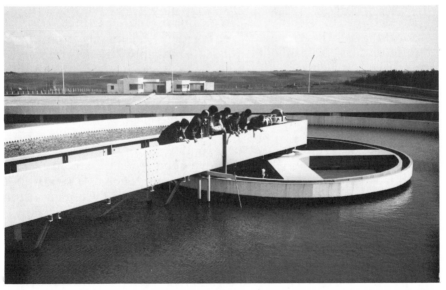

Water purification plant. It is far easier to pollute than to purify water, and man is finding it increasingly difficult and expensive to purify contaminated water for his own consumption. (Courtesy of the World Health Organization)

Biocides. Biocide is a term borrowed from Richard Wagner's *Environment and Man.* It is used instead of pesticide or insecticide because these two terms do not accurately describe those substances used to destroy a specific insect and yet also potentially injurious to other living things. No compound is available which will destroy only one pest while leaving unharmed other living things in the environment.

The most immediate effects of the indiscriminant use of biocides are the inevitable alterations of biological ecosystems and the development of resistant strains of the target organisms. Predators and prey are common to any ecosystem, and the elimination of one has profound effects on the other—overpopulation of the prey when the predator is eliminated and migration to more "fertile" areas by predators if the prey is destroyed. In either case the natural balance is destroyed, sometimes with disastrous effects to crops, to other wildlife, and occasionally to communities. In California, for example, over a million acres of cotton field were sprayed to destroy the lygus bug. The spray was toxic to a broad spectrum of other insects and eliminated most of them. The chemical did not persist and, in the absence of natural predators, lygus bugs moved back into the field and began reproducing rapidly. Repeated applications were required, increasing the likelihood that over a few seasons the lygus bug would become resistant to that particular biocide.

Resistance to biocides is becoming of increasing concern to community health officials. When a small percentage of an insect population survives a biocide attack, its multiplication is often more rapid than the original strain because it can reproduce without competition from its "peers" and often in the absence of its predators. Beginning in 1947 with the emergence of houseflies resistant to DDT, an increasing number of DDT-resistant insects has appeared including the malaria-carrying mosquito, lice, fleas, and a number of other disease vectors. In 1967 over 160 insect species formerly controlled by DDT had developed resistant strains. Compounding the problem is the occasional emergence of a strain that is not only resistant to a biocide but lives longer and produces more eggs than its predecessor.

Perhaps the most threatening problem of biocide use is a phenomenon called *biological magnification.* Some biocides, such as DDT, are highly soluble in fat and will accumulate in the cellular fat bodies of algae. Organisms eating the algae accumulate the biocide in higher concentrations and so on up the food chain to seriously damaging concentrations in birds, for example (see Figure 4.2). Man is at the top of many food chains and has accumulations of DDT in body fat. The effects of such accumulations are unknown

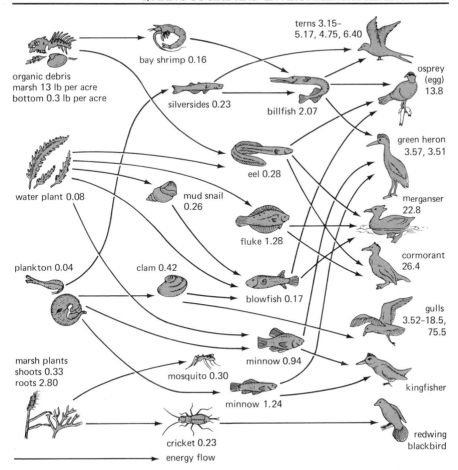

FIGURE 4.2. **Biological magnification. Note how the DDT concentration increases in the food chain of the estuarian biosphere shown here. The same process occurs for mercury and lead, but in different food chains.** [*From G. M. Woodwell, "Toxic Substances in Ecological Cycles,"* Scientific American, *216 (1967): 26*]

to the extent that no known incidences of sickness or death can be attributed to biocide accumulation. Deaths due to accidental intakes of biocides among agricultural workers have occurred, indicting these substances as poisonous. Whether biological magnification can in the long term produce a poisonous or other serious reaction in man is a chance we should not be willing to take.

Control of Environmental Health Problems

Because of the potential enormity of our collective pollution problems, a tremendous number of human, economic, and legislative resources have been brought to bear in these cases. Far-reaching legislative packages have been passed at all levels of government from the creation of the Federal Environmental Protection Agency to leaf-burning ordinances at the local level. While it is too early to judge the cumulative effects of these efforts over an extended period of time, it is evident that gains have been few in number and gradual in time. Emission-control devices on automobiles have done little to ease the air-pollution problem; lead-free gasoline has not been a large marketing success, although it has potential for reducing atmospheric pollution. Some water supples have been reclaimed while others have become contaminated. Some industries, mostly small ones, have effectively controlled waste disposal and particulate-matter release; others have effectively stalled any action at all. A few state and local control programs, such as sewage-treatment facilities, have been effective; others have been pigeon-holed by political or economic rationalizations. The net effect to date has been small steps where giant steps are required.

As stated earlier, the political, social, and economic ramifications of environmental problems and their solutions are enormously complex. The complexity itself is a major barrier to possible solutions since so many interrelated conditions have to be dealt with. Can a pollution-free automobile be manufactured that will be relatively inexpensive and marketable in terms of noise, appearance, and comfort? How much unemployment will it cause in the auto industry? How much retooling of manufacturing plants? Will the large oil lobbyists resist? Will the energy source for the automobile further deplete natural resources or produce other detrimental effects on the environment? And finally, will the trade-offs and possible sacrifices be willingly accepted by the population? Multiply the questions by the number of environmental problems and the results become almost overpowering to the man on the street.

Individual action to fight pollution is a vain hope even at the local level. Pollution knows no geographical or political boundaries and must be fought on a larger scale to be effective. Public policy, supported and enforced, must be the primary focus of attack if environmental problems are to be controlled. Individual action is best used to influence public policy and to ensure the adherence to those policies once implemented.

The first step, however, is a reeducation of large segments of our population. Cleaning up our environment and establishing quality rather than quantity as a goal of American life will require a redirecting of our technology, national standards of quality for the goods we produce, sweeping changes in the performance and goals of our institutions, and a reshaping of our values. But first and foremost, it will require of all people the development of an ecological ethic of understanding and respect for the bonds that unite man with the natural systems of the planet. Acceptance of this ethic will require nothing less than achieving a transition from a predominantly consumer society to one that respects its place among all elements of nature and concerns itself with the total well-being of present and future generations.

Educational approaches must be instituted that will effectively bring pollution problems closer to home, that is, will create in the average consumer and the local politician a feeling of responsibility for and indentification with a problem he faces now rather than, as often publicized, 50 years in the future. Our tendency to react to immediate problems is far stronger than our concern for preventing future ones. The need for man to "hold off" from gross and irreversible environmental destruction is no more immediate than now. The role of the community health professional in this reeducation process is crucial. He stands in a unique position, with avenues of influence not only to the consumer who shapes public policies but to the governmental bodies which must legislate them and the social and professional institutions which must support and implement them.

TOPICS FOR DISCUSSION

1. Discuss the reasons why the average consumer does not seem to be overly concerned with pollution problems. Do any of these reasons apply to any other diseases discussed in Chapters 3 and 4?
2. In relation to mental health, discuss the following statement: "Most drugs are designed to treat the patient's symptoms; the concept of cure is usually forgotten."

Part Two

The Study of Community Health Problems

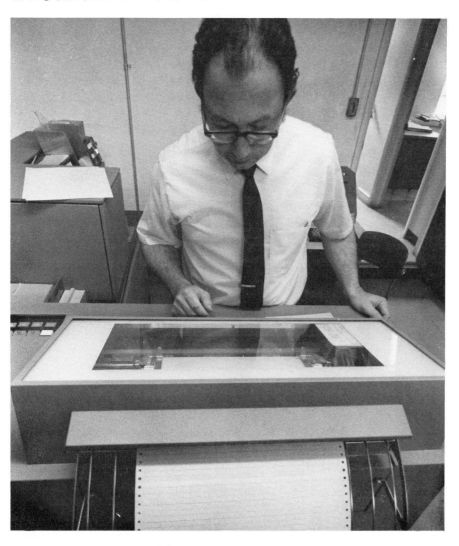

The large scale and long-term nature of many epidemiological studies necessitate computer-ized methods of data processing. *(Photo on previous page courtesy of the World Health Organization)*

5. The Science of Epidemiology

Public and community health practices came into being as a result of a fundamental need for the application of disease control methods to large groups of people. Unlike the medical clinician, the community health professional works in an ever-changing environment and without the benefit of precision and control so fundamental to the clinical sciences. His "laboratory" is the community and his "subjects" the population, both of which are dynamic and often unpredictable. His broad objective is to acquire sufficient knowledge of both community and population groups to be able to formulate measures for disease control and prevention. The public views the community health professional most commonly as a dispenser of services, an administrator of programs. Behind this public image, however, there exists a broad network of investigative techniques and procedures for the collection of vast amounts of data which, when analyzed, form the basis for nearly all other functions of the community health profession.

The effectiveness of community health practices depends on a thorough knowledge of the unique characteristics of any group of people, large or small, for from this knowledge comes an understanding of the disease processes and health problems which affect that community. Community health programs are successful only to the extent that they are designed to "fit" the population groups most affected by the specific health problems at hand. The study of community populations for the purpose of designing appropriate programs is fundamental to the community health profession, and the techniques and procedures by which it is accomplished are collectively referred to as the science of epidemiology.

THE MEANING OF EPIDEMIOLOGY

Epidemiology can be referred to as the "quiet science" of the community health profession, for few people are familiar with the term and the function of epidemiology and fewer yet can come close to its definition. Attempts to define it range from as far out as the "study of skin diseases" to the "study of epidemics." The latter definition is supported by modern dictionaries which define the term as "the branch of medicine dealing with epidemics and epidemic diseases." Such a definition represents a throwback to the late 1800s and early 1900s when the systematic study and control of communicable diseases occurring in epidemic form was just beginning. To study an epidemic meant to analyze its pattern of occurrence among population groups, and to the techniques and procedures of such analyses the term *epidemiology* was applied. For several decades, the science was devoted almost exclusively to communicable disease control—understandably so, for diseases such as pneumonia, influenza, and tuberculosis were the leading causes of death in this period.

To define contemporary epidemiology solely in terms of "epidemics," however, is to disregard a major portion of its functions and contributions to the study of modern health problems. The transition from the communicable diseases of earlier periods to the socially-based health problems of today represents a change from relatively simple disease processes to highly complex and multi-faceted health problems—a change which requires a broadening in scope of both the process and definition of epidemiology. This breadth is acknowledged in the following definition: epidemiology is *the applied science of the discovery and measurement of the circumstances under which health problems occur among groups of people.*

Within this definition, there are several key words and concepts which indicate the basic orientation of epidemiology. It is a *science* by virtue of its specialized techniques, measurement devices, language, and the quantitative information it contributes to the understanding and control of health problems. *Measurement* identifies the procedures for the accumulation and analysis of massive amounts of statistical data related to populations and disease conditions. *Circumstances under which health problems occur* refers to the many and complex variables that enter into the etiology of contemporary health problems, for the epidemiologist is concerned with the mental, social, behavioral, physical, and environmental aspects of community health problems. *Groups of people,* or populations, are the major targets of epidemiological investigations; little professional consideration is given to single instances of disease except as each may represent a potential source of information applicable to larger population groups who could suffer from the same disease condition.

The science of epidemiology provides a dimension to the study of health problems not provided by any of the other medical sciences. It can be distinguished from clinical-diagnostic procedures in that it seeks to discover patterns of disease occurrences: to whom these diseases occur and where and when they tend to flourish. Given the social nature of many of today's health problems, the clinical diagnosis and treatment of a single patient and the study of chemical and physiological characteristics of a particular health problem may reveal only a partial understanding of the problem. The true nature of drug addiction, mental illnesses, obesity, or similar present-day problems emerges only after repeated studies of the afflicted groups to identify the common characteristics of both the disease processes and the victims. Since life styles are major factors in disease causation, the discovery of the circumstances that distinguish those afflicted from the rest of the population may provide the most significant contribution to the prevention and control of a given health problem.

HISTORICAL DEVELOPMENT

In its broadest sense, epidemiology is a process of organized and purposeful observation. It is the product of man's persistent efforts to find cause-and-effect relationships among the forces and conditions surrounding disease and other health problems. As in all scientific disciplines, human curiosity is the basic motivation, and the emergence of epidemiology as a science was preceded by the sporadic but continued accumulation of knowledge and recorded observations over a span of many centuries. The history of medicine is in large measure a chronology of man's continual efforts to understand the causes of disease and epidemics by rational interpretation of the circumstances under which the problems occurred. Observation and the logical association of events provided the basis for the development of a wide variety of theories on disease causation, treatment, and prevention. Throughout history, man observed that disease and pestilence occurred in concert with changes in weather and seasons, movements of people, drought, famine, and other visible conditions. Relating these conditions to prevailing cultural and social ideologies, he developed over the centuries an impressive array of theories and cause-and-effect explanations: from demonism to the humoral theory to the existence of miasmatic vapors. As cultural and social ideologies changed—from religious to environmental concerns, for example—so, too, did the theories of disease causation. That many of these theories seem naive and even grotesque in light of modern medical knowledge in no way demeans the process by which they evolved. Modern medicine and the methods of disease control are no less dependent than their forebearers on the process of observation and the rational association of events. Unlike their historical counterparts, however, contemporary scientists have access to a vast store of scientific knowledge and information, a great deal of which owes its existence to the efforts and discoveries of the past.

The modern epidemiologist would do well to study in depth the history of his science. There is no better way to develop a sound appreciation for the observational process and a clear understanding of the fundamental importance of evaluating health problems in light of social and cultural forces. Religion, mysticism, superstition, ethnic origin, and cultural value systems continue to exert enormous influences on the health behavior of large segments of the population of any nation. For this reason, community health professionals generally and epidemiologists specifically can make their most significant contributions to medical science by describing accurately all the characteristics of specific populations that may relate to the occurrence of health problems and the effectiveness of health programs among those populations.

The Religious Era

Throughout history, of all cultural institutions religion has had the most fundamental effect on theories of disease causation and on the acceptable methods of treatment and prevention. All-powerful dieties were assumed to control the physical forces in man's environment, and thus they were believed to exert the controlling influence on his life and fate.

Primitive man explained and accepted the most catastrophic occurrences on the basis of reasonably simple observations of events and in conjunction with his religious beliefs. Good and evil spirits were believed responsible for prosperity and devastation, respectively. Natural occurrences such as flood, fire, earthquakes, and tidal waves were viewed as direct attempts by the evil spirits to wreak destruction upon mankind. Primitive man observed that natural disasters were often followed by epidemics, famine, and pestilence, and because of this association of events he attributed these aftermaths to the same evil spirits. Whether the diseases were inflicted upon one member of the tribe or epidemic to the entire population, the remedy was the same: appease the evil spirits or drive them out of the afflicted. Sacrifices, tribal rites, and incantations were the methods used to accomplish these ends, and all courses of action were decided by the tribal priest, the first of history's "medicine men." Thus evolved the most primitive form of disease control, emerging from simple observations of events which were then assimilated into the religious beliefs and cultural traditions of tribal societies. The priest or other religious representative of the tribe was established as the source of all counsel for matters of illness and disaster, a position of authority that was to last for many centuries—even to the present time in some cultures.

As man's religious thinking evolved and monotheism devel-

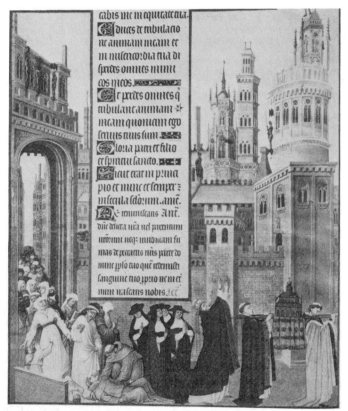

In medieval times, religious doctrines often shaped medical theories and practices. Epidemics were often attributed to the anger of God, and plague processions, such as the one pictured above, were conducted throughout the city and countryside to beg God to cease wreaking his vengeance. *(From the "Très Riches Heures" of the Duc de Berry. Musée Condé, Chantilly, and The New York Academy of Medicine)*

oped, disease and pestilence were perceived as retribution for transgressions of divine laws. Although demonism had abated, the primitive approach to the prevention and control of disease remained the same: appease the offended diety by making such offerings or atonements as the priest or church rituals prescribed. Under church domination, man so subjugated himself to his God that in the early Middle Ages his life style was devoted to the complete sacrifice of all but the most basic worldly goods. To live in poverty and filth and to reject all things worldly and material was the ultimate appeasement of a vengeful God. While such a life style was rejected by many, there can be little doubt that the great plagues of history were in part the result of squalid living conditions which in turn were the result of the near-complete domination of religious beliefs over those of a scientific or observational nature. To view disease as a product of man and his environment was to reject the basic religious doctrines of the time.

To this day, religion continues to exert a strong influence on individual decisions in matters of health and medicine. Beyond the persistent and sincere belief by many that spiritual rather than secular forces control the development of disease and ill-fortune, there lies the contemporary reappearance of mysticism, astrology, and demonism. The return of the evil spirit in modern trappings brings full circle the intimate relationship between religious beliefs and attitudes towards the cause and control of the misfortunes of life.

The Era of Physical Forces

While the Church's control over man's spiritual universe remained strong in the late Middle Ages and Renaissance, its influence on his physical environment decreased. As towns and cities began to grow and become more organized, the attributes of hard work and thrift and the adequate provision of food, clothing, and shelter became fundamental to the "good life." Since disease and pestilence were threats to this life, man began to search for more worldly explanations for their existence and control. It was believed that God's will could best be served on earth by living a good life reasonably free of the encumbrances of disease, and that to accomplish this goal man should attempt to control the forces of destruction around him—to turn his eyes away from the heavens and search the environment in which he lives. From this perspective a number of theories of disease causation began to emerge which were based on physical and environmental factors.

The transition from religious to secular considerations in

health matters resulted in a curious mixture of health practices and beliefs which have persisted in varying degrees to the present. Prayer, fasting, and sacrifices return in the face of severe disease problems that persist despite the application of scientific control measures. In colonial times, days of prayer were set aside during a smallpox epidemic in Boston, though the General Court wisely moved across the bay to Charlestown. Cotton Mather preached that disease was the avenging whip of God, but hastily added that his parishioners should make every effort to receive their innoculations. In 1832 President Jackson was petitioned to set aside a national day of prayer and fasting as a precaution against the spread of cholera which had appeared on the North Atlantic seaboard.

While undercurrents of religious theories persisted, the physical environment became the dominant focus of observation and investigation. Disease and pestilence became more closely associated with events in the environment—ranging from astrological movements of heavenly bodies to tidal variations to decay and filth. All such occurrences were carefully observed in conjunction with the incidence of disease in attempts to establish cause-and-effect relationships.

From the many theories that evolved, the predominant one was the theory of toxic miasmata and vapors, often referred to as the *miasmatic theory.* This theory held that disease resulted from poisons, vapors, and mists (miasma) that rose up from the earth or came in from the sea and were spread by the winds. Dating from Hippocrates in the pre-Christian era, the miasmatic theory provided a broad and fitting basis for the assimilation of theories of disease causation with existing beliefs. The position of heavenly bodies, tidal movements, decay and filth, fog and swamp gases —each occurrence through observation could offer an acceptable explanation for the origin of miasmatic mists and vapors. Coastal areas were at the mercy of tides and fog coming in from the sea; crowded city populations were constantly exposed to the atmospheric effects of filth, sewage, and decaying matter; people residing near swamps and marshes breathed the vapors and gases emanating from them. For all diseases, individual or epidemic, a convenient and observable explanation was now available.

Man's attention was now directed towards his environment and his powers of observation were used to establish, however unsoundly, cause-and-effect relationships. The science of epidemiology can trace its origin to this period of history when it became commonplace to relate environmental circumstances to the major epidemic diseases of the day. That people living near swamps were found to have a high incidence of fevers was explained by the exist-

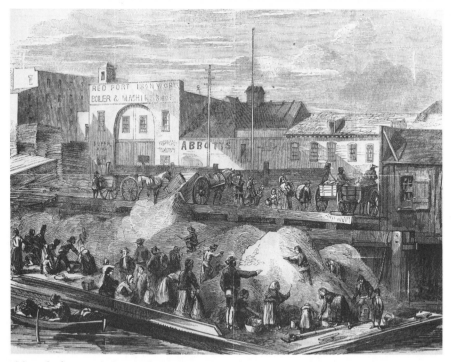

Although the association made in the nineteenth century between filth and the spread of disease was valid, it was based incorrectly on the belief that poisonous vapors (miasma) emanating from the decaying matter were the cause of illness. This theory of disease causation did little to relieve the disease-ridden poor, however. The above is a dumping ground at the foot of Beach Street in New York City in 1866; as soon as refuse was thrown onto the barge, the poor were there ready to pick through it. *(National Library of Medicine, Bethesda, Maryland)*

ence of swamp gases. The surrounding air was made bad by these gases, and the fever came to be known as malaria (*mal aria*—"bad air"). The spread of epidemics and pestilence throughout the crowded, poorer sections of cities was attributed to toxic emanations of decaying filth. In 1793 Benjamin Rush attributed an outbreak of yellow fever to the decay of a shipload of coffee that had piled up on the wharves. Outbreaks of typhoid and cholera were said to be caused by defective house drains and the rise and fall of ground water.

Attempts to control these disease conditions were logical outgrowths of the theory. "Cleaning the air" of poisonous elements was attempted by firing cannons and building fires in the town square, by fumigating and burning homes and buildings thought to be polluted. Ships on which disease victims traveled were often punctured to let out the poisonous gases and then sometimes burned in the harbor. Filth removal campaigns also became prominent. As early as 1797, a Massachusetts statute empowered a board of health to regulate "dangerous and noisome odors" and "to control sources of filth and causes of disease." Philadelphia attempted to prevent an invasion of cholera in 1832 by a program of municipal cleanliness. In 1850, after conducting an extensive investigation of the health problems in Boston, Lemuel Shattuck presented his famous "Report to the Sanitary Commission of Massachusetts," a remarkable document that served as an early prototype for the basic functions and objectives of public health departments. In it Shattuck not only recommended the establishment of state and local boards of health but also urged the initiation of regular and systematic sanitary inspections, census-takings, food and drug control, studies of health problems related to housing and air pollution and to special population groups such as immigrants and school children, and periodic and routine physical examinations for private citizens to promote the prevention of disease.

Along with Shattuck, other prominent names in the historical evolution of modern medicine and epidemiology emerged from the nineteenth century. Ignatz Semmelweiss made the audacious suggestion that doctors wash their hands before examining obstetrical cases to remove the infectious material which he had deduced to be the cause of puerperal, or childbed, fever. It·remained for Oliver Wendell Holmes several years later to gather additional evidence to substantiate this relationship. Peter Ludwig Panum studied a serious outbreak of measles on the Faroe Islands in 1846 and established many of the basic facts about the nature of the disease. During a cholera outbreak in one section of London in 1849, John Snow noted a definite pattern between the people who drank the water from one particular well and those who came down with the disease. By simply removing the handle of the pump, he was able to arrest the spread of cholera that year. The contributions of these early practitioners are even more remarkable in light of the fact that the existence of microscopic life had not yet been discovered.

The theory of toxic miasmata and vapors did a great deal to advance the process of sanitation and the control of environmental causes and spread of infectious diseases, even though it offered an unsound explanation of the true origin of the diseases. More importantly, however, it brought about an attitude, a state of mind, that both provoked and permitted the bacteriological discoveries that followed. In addition, it demonstrated the value of studying "populations" of disease victims to discover common experiences and exposure to environmental conditions—the basic process of epidemiology.

Bacteriological Era

While many people like John Snow were investigating certain environmental conditions as sources of disease, Louis Pasteur was carrying out his now-famous studies of the existence and pathogenic nature of microscopic life. Before the end of the nineteenth century, he had shown conclusively that bacterial organisms were indeed virulent to man and that they arose from self-propagation, not spontaneously from the environment. Life arises from preexisting life, even in microscopic form.

Even though Pasteur's evidence was beyond scientific dispute, old ideas and theories die hard. The miasmatic theory provided paradoxical but firm opposition to the emerging germ theory of disease. Man's strength of observation and rational association of

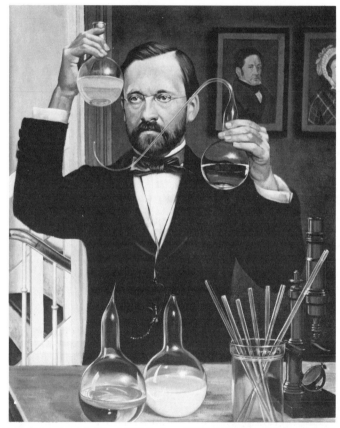

Through careful experimentation, Louis Pasteur (1822–1895) was able to prove that microbial organisms are reproduced from parent organisms and not through spontaneous generation. His further demonstration of their pathogenic nature was to transform medical practice. *(Courtesy of Parke, Davis & Company, © 1962)*

observable events, so well established under the miasmatic theory, now seemed to be challenged by the existence of mysterious forces that could not be observed or studied without the use of scientific gadgets called microscopes. That man, the highest form of life, could be brought to his knees by an invisible bit of primitive matter seemed beyond the power of imagination. Inexorably, however, the evidence mounted as additional pathogens were identified and proven to be the cause of specific disease conditions. Animals and insects were recognized as hosts and carriers, and the search for environmental sources of bacterial growth was intensified. Programs of sanitation, fumigation, and disinfection, originating under the miasmatic theory, were continued but directed specifically at known and suspected areas of bacterial contamination and sources of the spread of infection.

Amid nearly militant opposition, the germ theory of disease was firmly established by the end of the nineteenth century. One discovery was yet to be made, however, before the epidemiological picture of infectious diseases could be completed and the miasmatic theory laid to rest. In 1912 Charles V. Chapin published *The Sources and Modes of Infection* in which he clearly established the predominance of man over environment as the primary reservoir or source of pathogenic life. With a few major exceptions, as in the cases of tuberculosis, typhoid, and intestinal diseases, pathogenic organisms cannot survive in the inanimate environment but require the life-supporting elements that only living tissue can provide. With this discovery, all avenues for the complete investigation of infectious diseases were known and available for intensive study. The establishment of the pathogenic agent, the human (or animate) host, and the environment as elements common to all communicable diseases marks the point in history when epidemiology began its transformation from an informal observational process to the scientific study of epidemics. The discovery of the processes by which diseases spread and flourish became the unique domain of the epidemiological method, and from the persistent application of evolving principles of investigation emerged the classical trilogy of the epidemiological analysis of communicable diseases.

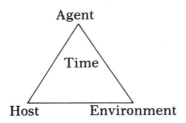

This traditional model represents not only the basic structure for the study of communicable diseases but also the birth of epidemiology as a science. The growth of the science during the early decades of the twentieth century was marked by the development of data-gathering techniques, statistical representations and analysis of data, population sampling procedures, and case-finding and tracking techniques. Uniform legislation was passed creating state and local health departments, developing strict procedures for the reporting and publishing of vital health data, strengthening environmental sanitation procedures, and enforcing the application of preventive techniques emerging from the laboratory discoveries of immunologists and pharmacologists. Universities began to establish curricula for this new, specialized area of professional training.

Man's powers of observation and analysis were now armed with the language, techniques, and specificity of a science. Together with all other medical sciences, the application of epidemiological methods produced successes so astounding that by the middle of this century communicable diseases no longer dominated the mortality figures of the advanced societies of the world.

It is important to remember that epidemiology is the study of disease conditions as they occur among groups of people. In the recounting of events in the Bacteriological Era, specific discoveries of a clinical or laboratory nature tend to be singled out as dominant factors in the control of communicable diseases. As important as these discoveries were and continue to be, their value is limited by their specificity, by their application to particular organisms and disease conditions. To the community health profession, the immense significance of the Bacteriological Era goes beyond the discovery of particular causes and cures of certain diseases to the establishment of epidemiological methods and techniques broadly applicable to all populations and to all health conditions, regardless of their etiology.

Era Of Social Etiology

As discussed in earlier chapters, the steady decline of communicable diseases throughout this century brought to prominence other types of health problems that did not respond to the well-established techniques of clinical medicine, immunology, and sanitation. In the late 1940s the so-called diseases of civilization—the chronic and degenerative diseases—began to dominate the health and disease statistics, and they continue to do so today. Recently, health problems of a more insidious nature, long recognized but of lesser concern historically, have become headline material: drug abuse, social

alienation, alcoholism, psychosomatic illnesses, and ecological deg-
radation. In nearly all cases, social and behavioral factors play
dominant roles in the causation of these current health problems.

In view of this relatively new and complex influence of human
behavior on major health problems, the role of epidemiology has
been forced to expand in both importance and scope. The basic
flexibility of established epidemiological procedures, however, allowed for immediate adaptation from one set of health problems to
another. The classic trilogy needs to be modified only slightly to
represent the expanded role of the science.

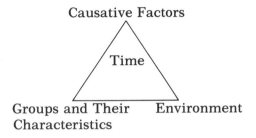

The change from Agent to Causative Factors is a reflection of
the shift from the search for a single causative agent to the identification of the multiple causes of modern health problems. Groups
and Their Characteristics replaces Host in the model in recognition
of the need to study modern health problems by identifying the
common demographic characteristics of those who fall victim to
these disease conditions. Developing a typical profile of heart attack
victims by age, race, sex, education, personal habits, and so forth,
provides the type of information necessary in establishing preventive measures and identifying potential victims of heart attacks.
The term Environment remains the same, although it now connotes
a more comprehensive association among the social, ecological,
behavioral, as well as physical elements in the relationship of people to their surroundings.

The expansion of epidemiology into social and behavioral areas
has been a relatively easy transition but not without its problems
and frustrations. In retrospect, the problems of infectious diseases
were simple puzzles that were solved for the most part by the application of knowledge and medications derived primarily through
laboratory discoveries. In comparison, today's health problems are
made infinitely more complex by the absence of specific causitive
factors and the presence of the complications of human behavior.
The modern epidemiologist is not unlike Semmelweiss, Snow, and
Panum who nearly a century ago sought solutions to perplexing

disease problems by searching the population and environment for common denominators in the disease process.

In modern times, the community health profession has reached out into other disciplines for accumulation of data and expert counsel. Many population studies related to health problems and behavior are being conducted in the social sciences, often in conjunction with health professions. Epidemiological investigations of drug usage, mental illnesses, sexual deviations, psychosomatic ailments, and a wide variety of other disorders are being conducted by sociologists, political scientists, psychologists, ecologists, and educators. Terms such as "social epidemiology," "public health sociology," "social medicine," and "medical ecology" are becoming commonplace in the literature of these related professions. The immediate trend in the science of epidemiology is toward the interdisciplinary pooling of resources, manpower, data, and expertise in order to investigate and analyze more effectively the health problems of today.

THE EPIDEMIOLOGICAL PROCESS

The primary purpose of the epidemiological study of a health problem is to describe and analyze the common characteristics of a particular problem and of the populations affected by it. To accomplish this purpose, procedures and instruments are devised to collect data which pertain to specific characteristics of the people affected by the problem and to its variations of occurrence according to time and place. Not all studies will seek data in all three areas, however. Some may single out place, for example, to fill in missing data or to test more stringently the hypothesis that geographical location is a primary factor in the occurrence or causation of a particular disease.

Characteristics of People

Subjects in epidemiological studies are most commonly profiled, or described, according to such variables as age, sex, ethnic origin, occupation, and education. However, other variables may be included if the investigator has reason to believe that other factors may be relevant to the study. Religion, socioeconomic level, marital status, history of specific diseases, immunization records, and so forth, are not uncommon categories in some of the more specialized epidemiological investigations.

Age is perhaps the most significant variable, and its association with particular health problems has been the most frequently noted.

Age patterns of certain diseases have been so well established that constant references are made to "childhood diseases" and "diseases of the elderly." The medical specialties of pediatrics and geriatrics give further evidence of the importance of the age-related nature of diseases.

Sex and ethnic origin are also important variables in the description of the pattern of many diseases. Illness and death rates often reveal significant differences between men and women and between white and nonwhite populations. These differences are reflected in Figure 5.1, which compares the mortality rates of these groups. Diseases such as lung cancer and heart disease are more likely to occur in men than in women. Hypertensive heart disease, tuberculosis, and pneumonia occur more often among nonwhite

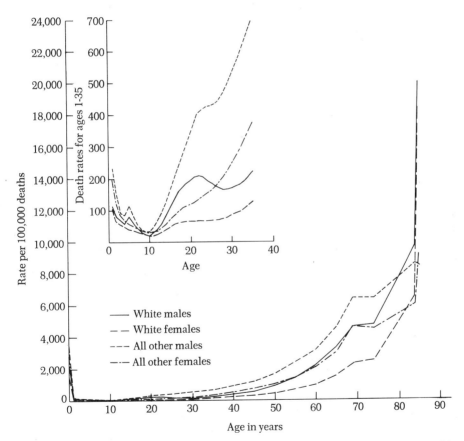

FIGURE 5.1.   Death rates by age, sex, and color: United States, 1969. (U.S. Public Health Service)

populations, while arteriosclerotic heart disease and suicide are more common among whites.

Characteristics of Time

Time often proves to be a crucial factor in the control of specific health problems, and the investigation of disease patterns according to time can reveal significant and specific fluctuations in occurrence or symptoms. Incubation periods may be short or long, seasonal variations may occur, disease complications may appear at particular intervals, epidemics such as influenza can occur in cyclical patterns, or disease problems may change in number and intensity as social patterns change. Knowledge of these temporal variations can be extremely useful in the prevention of particular diseases or in the control of the course of a disease once it has started. The relevant time period (year, season, days, hours of the day, and so forth) will vary according to the health problem under consideration.

Changes occurring over long periods of time are known as *secular changes.* A great deal of data related to mortality and morbidity is collected every year for purposes of comparing present information with that collected during past years. Figure 5.2 gives two examples of secular change. Progress in medical science and health care is in part measured through such comparisons. Statistics on

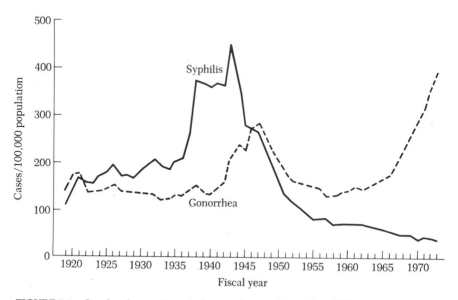

FIGURE 5.2.   Secular change. Reported cases of gonorrhea and syphilis per 100,000 population by year: United States, 1919–1973. *(Center for Disease Control, U.S. Public Health Service)*

secular changes also provide information on alterations in disease patterns and fluctuations in the severity of certain diseases.

Short-term fluctuations in disease patterns are most often described as *seasonal* and *cyclic changes* and *point epidemics.* Seasonal incidences of diseases are often clearly identifiable not only in instances of infectious disease but also in cases of accidents, such as drownings in the summertime. Malaria and bacillary dysentery are more prevalent in the hot months in most parts of the world. During the winter months, upper respiratory diseases and measles are common; diphtheria and scarlet fever reach their peak in the autumn; mumps, rubella, and whooping cough are more common in the springtime. As seen in Figure 5.3, salmonella (food poisoning) is significantly more prevalent during the summer months.

Cyclic changes, or cycles of disease, refer to the predictable occurrence of diseases by spans of years. Scarlet fever occurs in five-year cycles, measles in three-year cycles, and meningococcal meningitis every eight to ten years. These cyclic patterns are generally characteristic of infectious diseases and have been modified somewhat by the use of antibiotics and vaccines.

The main characteristic of a point epidemic is its explosiveness—the sudden outbreak of a large number of cases in a matter of hours or days. Such a rash of cases usually points to a single source of infection, such as contaminated food, radiation

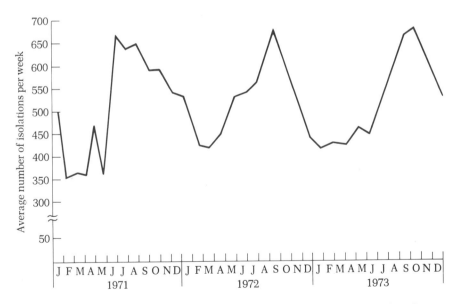

FIGURE 5.3.   Seasonal change. Surveillance program isolations of salmonella from humans per month: United States, 1971–1973. *(Center for Disease Control, U.S. Public Health Service)*

leakage, or polluted water. John Snow in his investigation of a cholera outbreak in London plotted the occurrence of the disease as
shown in Figure 5.4. The large number of cases occurring during
late August identifies this outbreak as a classic point epidemic.
Other common diseases that often follow a similar pattern are food
poisoning, milk-borne typhoid fever, chemical poisoning, and ali-
mentary diseases such as bacillary dysentery.

There are additional circumstances in which time becomes an
important element in the description of disease patterns. The possibility of german measles in the mother causing birth defects in her
baby is much greater during the second month of pregnancy than
at any other time during pregnancy. Figure 5.5 illustrates the importance of time as related to the incubation period of serum hepatitis.
That as many as 135 days can elapse between exposure and the
appearance of symptoms is a crucial piece of clinical information.

Characteristics of Place

Geographical units of varying types and sizes are used in the
description of geographical patterns of disease. It is common to
compare death and disease rates among nations of the world, states,
regions of the United States, and the smaller segments such as cities,
townships, and census tracts. Maps such as that shown in Figure 5.6
are the most commonly used in presenting this type of data. Other
geographical units are used but with less frequency. For example,
to study the effects of fluoridated water requires the use of popula-

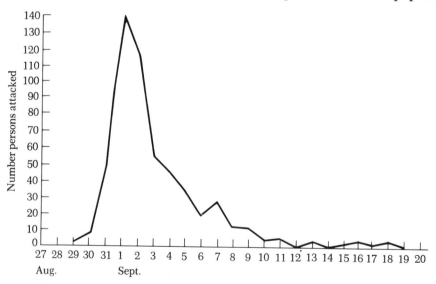

FIGURE 5.4.   Point epidemic. Cholera outbreak in London, August–September 1848.

tions with such a supply of water and a comparable population with unfluoridated water. High altitude conditions have been studied for a possible connection with rheumatic fever and rheumatoid arthritis. Some soil and water conditions may have a relationship to certain cardiovascular diseases. A current trend in "social epidemiology" is comparative studies between urban and rural populations, inner-city and suburban groups, and residents of economically depressed areas and the well-to-do residential sections of the country. While the focus in these studies is on people, the effect of their geographical locations must be taken fully into account.

The interaction between people and their environment often makes it difficult to study geographical units and their specific relationship to health problems. Boundaries of living space, such as city or state lines, are established for political rather than health reasons. Since most health problems do not have such boundaries, geographical demarcations often place artificial and misleading limitations on the effective study of these problems. In addition, the people living in certain geographical units are sufficiently different from other population groups to make comparative studies by geog-

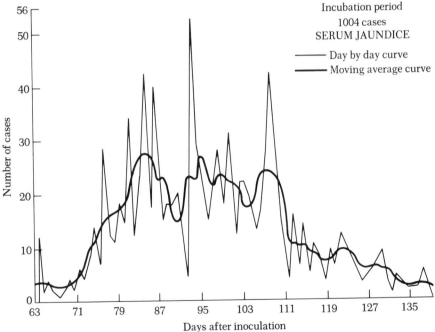

FIGURE 5.5. Variable incubation periods were responsible for the prolonged outbreak of serum hepatitis among 1,004 men in a military camp who were inoculated at the same time with the same dose of the same lot of vaccine. *(Reprinted from* Clinical Epidemiology *by John R. Paul by permission of The University of Chicago Press. Copyright 1958)*

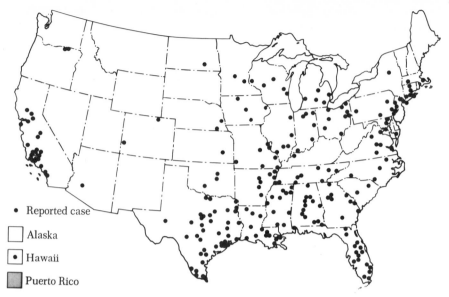

FIGURE 5.6.   Geographic distribution. Reported cases of tetanus: United States, 1950–1966. *(From* Annual Supplement, Summary 1966. *Atlanta: National Communicable Disease Center, 1967)*

raphy very difficult. Care must be exercised to ensure at least a gross similarity between population groups before such comparisons can be made with any degree of validity. Many differences in disease occurrence according to geographical location are influenced by such factors as rainfall, climate, soil and water characteristics, and the cultural, social, and economic characteristics of the local population.

THE USES OF EPIDEMIOLOGY

Epidemiology is only one of the fundamental sciences related to the fields of medicine and community health. It stands alone in the study of health problems among groups of people, but it contributes little to the clinical relationship between the doctor and his patient, the microbiologist and his laboratory studies, and the physiologist and his experimental research. This perspective is perhaps best stated by John R. Paul, noted epidemiologist: "The epidemiological method is the only way of asking some questions, one way of asking others, and no way at all to ask many."[1]

In the history of the modern world, the scientific contributions of epidemiology and the uses of its methodology have been so great as to place it near the forefront of the extensive effort to control the health problems of the day. The modern emphasis on the prevention of disease and the concentration on the "why" rather than the "how" of health problems depend on the type of data that only the methods of epidemiology can provide. The important contributions of this science to the health and medical professions can best be described by considering the broad range of uses to which epidemiological information can be applied.

(1) *To study the history of a health problem specifically or the health of populations generally.* The alterations in disease patterns and severity provide the data from which future trends can be established and preventive action taken. For example, the cyclic variations of diseases such as influenza and measles have been identified by careful measurement of epidemics of them occurring during the last five decades. The patterns established provide the basis for predictions of future epidemics and allow ample time to prepare treatment and preventive programs. In some instances, the study of disease patterns provides data which form the only basis for the successful prevention of a given disease. For example, very little is known about the etiology of rheumatic fever, and little can be done to prevent complications such as rheumatic heart disease. Epidemiological studies of the disease have revealed an established pattern of occurrence, however. As shown in Figure 5.7, rheumatic fever is often preceded by untreated cases of severe throat infection. There-

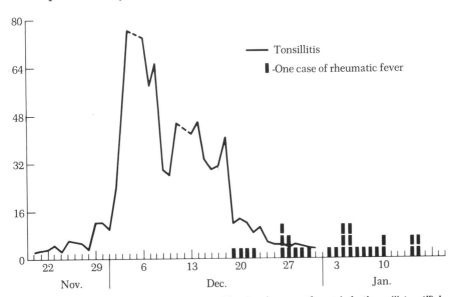

FIGURE 5.7. Pattern of occurrence. An epidemic of severe throat infections ("strept") in Denmark in 1926 was associated with or followed by an epidemic of rheumatic fever. *(Reprinted from* Clinical Epidemiology *by John R. Paul by permission of The University of Chicago Press. Copyright 1958)*

fore, the primary clinical procedure for the prevention of rheumatic fever is the antibiotic treatment of severe sore throats.

(2) *To diagnose the health of the community by developing health and disease profiles of population groups.* Population profiles of a given community are constructed from demographic data such as age, marital status, educational levels, occupation, and so forth. Such data often provide the epidemiologist with information sufficient to justify health programs that fit the population characteristics. An unusually large number of elderly, unemployed, or economically disadvantaged people in the population warrant the implementation of health services to meet the needs of these groups. Data concerning, for example, the number of people who smoke, are overweight, have high blood pressure, are not immunized, or are exposed to polluted air can be used to determine epidemiological profiles of disease potential in a population. From epidemiological data, the dimensions of health problems can be established for nearly any community or demographic group and specific services can be designed to fit specific populations. As life styles change, continuous investigation can reveal changes in health problems.

(3) *To study the effectiveness of health services and programs.* Health care services need constant evaluation to ensure that they are meeting the needs and demands of the community populations, and their effectiveness and efficiency can be measured for such an evaluation. For example, determining the levels of immunization in a population is a means of testing the effectiveness of immunization programs. A change in the infant mortality rate in a community is a measure of the success or failure of a well-baby clinic. Increases in the number of pap smears conducted reflect the success of a cancer education program.

(4) *To establish indices and estimations as to the individual risk or statistical probability of disease, injury, or accident.* To compile profiles of types of individuals prone to specific health problems is fundamental to epidemiological investigations. Drunken drivers, for example, are more likely to be involved in car accidents than are sober ones. The profile of a potential heart-attack victim is an individual who is male, is overweight, smokes, is hypertensive, and does not exercise. Such an epidemiological profile of high-risk individuals for a particular health problem can be derived only from data drawn from the population afflicted with that problem.

(5) *To complete the clinical picture of a disease.* Population data are added to medical, diagnostic, and laboratory information to provide complete descriptions of disease entities. The clinical picture of venereal diseases, for example, has been complete for many years, but the epidemiological data supplied the social and

cultural information that was vital to a complete understanding of these diseases.

(6) *To identify syndromes or combinations of symptoms that characterize a specific disease.* While gathering clinical information is not often the function of epidemiological studies, on occasion the description of relationships between people and their environment can provide this type of information. Studies of specific populations may reveal consistent symptoms of ill-health not recognized before. Studies of workers in plants manufacturing asbestos found that they had an abnormally high incidence of emphysema and lung cancer resulting from inhalation of asbestos filaments over a period of years. The symptoms of serum hepatitis among drug users was noted by epidemiological investigations and subsequently verified by clinical means.

SUMMARY

The basic purpose of the community health profession is to study health problems as they occur among population groups and to design effective control and preventive programs. Requisite to fulfilling this purpose is the study of populations to evaluate the conditions surrounding a given health problem and to seek clues as to its severity and scope. The techniques and procedures for carrying out such studies are the primary tools of the science of epidemiology.

The history of the science of epidemiology is a development of man's ability to observe the circumstances surrounding epidemics in an attempt to identify cause-and-effect relationships. The earliest primitive civilizations observed the association between natural disasters and the occurrences of disease and famine and, assigning a religious significance to it, they attempted through tribal rites and incantations to dissuade a vengeful deity from wreaking such punishments. As more civilized cultures evolved, man began to search his environment for the causes of disease and pestilence and formulated a number of theories as to the physical causation of epidemics. The most popular theory and the one which had the greatest influence on the development of epidemiological procedures was the miasmatic theory. While the theory itself was not valid, it brought about methods of sanitation and environmental control which are still in effect today. In addition, man's observation of environmental conditions laid the groundwork for his accepting the discoveries of microbial disease agents made by Pasteur and other bacteriologists and the eventual implementations of programs based on these discoveries for the control of infectious diseases. It remained only for Chapin to demonstrate that man is the primary reservoir for pathogens in order for the epidemiological picture of communicable diseases to be complete. At this point in the early 1920s, epidemiology changed from an informal observational process to an applied science. The application of its principles played a major role in the control of communicable diseases and continues to be of great importance in the study of today's more socially related health problems.

Contemporary epidemiologists study health problems by describing and analyzing them as they are related to specific population groups. The characteristics of people such as age, sex, and educational levels are identified; the effects of time on the duration and the intensity of the problems are studied; and geographical patterns of the occurrence of disease are evaluated—all of these data are analyzed to seek those elements which might be significant to the identification and description of the true nature of the health problems.

In view of our contemporary emphasis on the prevention of diseases and of the social nature of many of today's health problems, the science of epidemiology may prove to be the most significant force in the eventual control of these problems.

REFERENCES

1. John R. Paul, *Clinical Epidemiology* (Chicago: University of Chicago Press, 1966), p. 50.

TOPICS FOR DISCUSSION

1. In the recent past, epidemiology has been defined as the study of epidemics. Discuss the reasons why this definition no longer represents the true nature of the science of epidemiology.
2. Discuss the following statement: "The programs developed for the control of epidemics during the Era of Physical Forces resulted in the right actions but for the wrong reasons."
3. From current community health literature, select at least one epidemiological study that would illustrate the six uses of epidemiology discussed in this chapter.
4. Assume an outbreak of salmonella infections occurred in your local community. Using the principles of epidemiological investigations, how would you go about determining the source of the epidemic?

6. The Tools and Techniques of Epidemiology

As we saw in Chapter 5, the basic objective of epidemiology is to study the extent and intensity of a disease or health problem as it occurs among groups of people. To fulfill this objective involves the gathering of supportive, circumstantial evidence from which logical deductions can be made concerning cause, occurrence, treatment, and programming. With the community as his laboratory, the epidemiologist tries to determine the common factors associated with the occurrence of the health problems, such as place of occurrence, characteristics of the population affected, duration of the condition, and the specific nature of the health problem.

The skillful application of measurement and data-gathering techniques and the ability to analyze and draw logical inferences from the statistical information gathered are required of epidemiologists to fulfill this basic objective. The methods by which they collect data are many and varied, but for convenience can be classified according to the purpose of the investigation. To determine the specific characteristics of a population that are pertinent to a health problem a *descriptive study* is conducted; to develop hypotheses on the causes of a specific disease an *analytical study* is designed; and to determine the specific cause or causes of a given condition an *experimental study* is undertaken. The main difference among these types of studies is the extent to which conclusions about cause-and-effect relationships can be drawn—from severe limitations in descriptive data to positive proof in experimental studies.

DESCRIPTIVE STUDIES

"Counting heads" is perhaps the simplest definition of a descriptive study: the number of people with lung cancer who are heavy smokers, the number of females under the age of 35 in Hoboken, New Jersey, with lung cancer who smoke more than two packs of cigarettes per day. This is data-gathering in its most basic form, restricted to the enumeration of a specific number of population characteristics. As indicated by the figures throughout this and the previous chapter, the combinations of characteristics measured are infinite and are determined by the extent to which the investigator wishes to restrict the population being studied.

Whatever combination of data is used, the purpose of a descriptive study is to provide a clear, statistical picture of a public health problem. It provides the data by which the epidemiologist can determine, for example, the extent of an epidemic, the pattern of disease in terms of when, where, and to whom it occurs, the comparative change in disease rates over the years, the identification of "at-risk," or susceptible, populations, and so forth. In a descriptive study, conclusions must be limited to the specific "heads counted"—that is, the epidemiologist must preface his conclusions with such phrases as "in this specific sample," or "among those studied." In a single descriptive study the investigator cannot go beyond the actual numerical count obtained by his study. It would be improper and misleading to apply descriptive results to any other population group (one cannot conclude, for example, that if the immunization rate for measles for preschool children in Chicago is 65 percent, the rate would be similar in nearby suburban Lake Forest) or to assume a causal relationship between characteristics (one cannot infer from the fact that 65 percent of the pneumonia patients in a particular city last year were female that women in general must be more susceptible than men to pneumonia). Rarely does circumstantial evidence provide the basis for strong conclusions of a generalized nature. In practice, however, it is occasionally necessary in the face of severe health problems or overwhelming circumstantial data to assume a cause-and-effect relationship and act accordingly; John Snow's removal of the pump handle and the antismoking campaigns are good examples. The abuses of descriptive data, however, far outnumber the positive results of such conclusions. The phrase "you can prove anything with statistics" has its most common application in those situations where descriptive data are used to "prove" the cause of a health problem, the value of a medicine, the deleterious effects of substances or behaviors, and so forth. Judicious use of descriptive data demands not only the skill of measurement and the careful selection of the population characteristics to be measured, but also strict adherence to the limited interpretations possible from such data.

Presentation of Descriptive Data

Since "head-counting" is the basic procedure of descriptive epidemiology, data are always presented as raw numbers or their arithmetic derivatives (means, ratios, percentages and so on). Comparisons of data collected in different subject areas are often made to provide evidence of possible relationships and trends in disease patterns. The increasing parallel over the past few decades between lung cancer and cigarette smoking, the higher incidence of leukemia among the white population in the United States, the year-by-year decline in active cases of tuberculosis—all are numerical relationships developed by descriptive studies, and each adds substantially to our understanding of the nature of these health problems.

There are inherent problems in the use of numerical data, particularly when the populations studied are large. People have difficulty grasping large numbers representing populations. Large numbers often become abstractions, with the result that 5,000 deaths from a certain disease could sometimes take on greater enormity than 150,000 deaths from some other disease. In addition, it is impossible to make valid comparisons from raw numbers because population differences are not accounted for in simple numerical data.

For these reasons, descriptive statistics are most often converted to *rates.* Numerical data are broken down in such a way that the occurrence of death or disease can be presented in relationship to a standardized number of people—for example, 9.2 deaths per 1,000 in the population, 19.4 cases of cancer per 10,000 in the population, and so on. In the presentation of health data, a variety of rates is used. Each rate provides a different type of information, but all are based on the same principle and use a similar formula:

$$\frac{\text{Number of events for a given time period}}{\text{Population group}} \times 1,000; \ 10,000; \ \text{or } 100,000$$

An example of how this formula would be used is:

$$\frac{\text{Number of heart attacks in April 1975}}{\text{American males, white, ages 55–65}} \times 1,000$$

Types of Rates

Crude Rate. When it is desirable to express health data about an entire population, a *crude rate* is used. This rate is calculated without regard to population characteristics and includes all people in a specific geographic area. For example, the crude death rate in the United States for 1975 would be expressed as:

$$\frac{\text{Number of deaths in U.S. in 1975}}{\text{Midyear population of U.S.}} \times 10,000$$

The crude death rate for the state of Illinois would substitute Illinois data for U.S. data in the formula above. Crude rates have little practical value, and comparisons of crude rates are unreliable unless the population characteristics of two groups are similar. For example, if there were a higher number of elderly in Illinois than Indiana, the crude death rate in Illinois would be expected to be higher. Or, since death rates among nonwhites are generally higher than among the white population, comparisons of a predominantly white population with a predominantly nonwhite group would be highly misleading.

Nonetheless, crude rates are used to compare health data among large population groups, such as rates of cancer incidence in the United States and Russia, or the death rates in the United States in 1930 and 1970. Such comparisons are tenuous at best unless adjusted for population differences. Perhaps the greatest value of crude rates is their use as a general indicator of the extent of health-related events at a given time for large, heterogeneous populations.

Population-Specific Rates. The type of data that has the greatest application and is most commonly used in epidemiological studies is that which is broken down into specific population groups according to such characteristics as age, sex, race, education, and occupation. These population characteristics are called *demographic variables,* and population groups such as women, blacks, school children, and so forth are called *demographic groups.* The rates applied are called *population-specific rates.* For example, the mortality rate for females during 1975 would be calculated as follows:

$$\frac{\text{Sex-specific}}{\text{mortality rate}} = \frac{\text{Number of female deaths (1975)}}{\text{Midyear population of females (1975)}} \times 1,000$$

Rates for other demographic groups can be similarly drawn, and a large variety of combinations can be used at the discretion of the investigator to obtain more specific data. Commonly used rates are shown in Table 6.1.

Population-specific rates are valuable because they describe health events as they relate to population groups such as men, in-

TABLE 6.1   Measurements and indices commonly used in epidemiology

Age-specific death rate	$\dfrac{\text{Number of persons of a given age dying during the year}}{\text{Population in specified age group at midyear}}$	X 1000
Case-fatality rate	$\dfrac{\text{Number of deaths from a specified disease}}{\text{Number of cases of that disease}}$	X 100
Crude birth rate	$\dfrac{\text{Number of live births during the year}}{\text{Population at midyear}}$	X 1000
Crude death rate	$\dfrac{\text{Number of deaths occurring during the year}}{\text{Population at midyear}}$	X 1000
Infant death rate	$\dfrac{\text{Number of deaths of children under 1 year of age during the year}}{\text{Number of live births during that year}}$	X 1000
Maternal (puerperal) death rate	$\dfrac{\text{Number of deaths from puerperal causes during the year}}{\text{Number of live births during that year}}$	X 10000
Neonatal death rate	$\dfrac{\text{Number of deaths of children under 28 days of age during the year}}{\text{Number of live births during that year}}$	X 1000
Perinatal death rate	$\dfrac{\text{Number of fetal deaths and infant deaths under 7 days of age during the year}}{\text{Number of live births and fetal deaths during that year}}$	X 1000

fants, blue-collar workers, urban residents, and so on. Such data can be compared among all similar segments of any population group. The combinations of data are much too numerous for presentation here, but the examples presented in the Tables and Figures in this chapter demonstrate both the versatility and the value of simple descriptive studies.

ANALYTICAL STUDIES

Analytical studies are designed to go one step beyond descriptive investigations in an attempt to develop and test more specific hypotheses concerning the nature of specific disease problems. Descriptive data often provide clues about the cause of a particular health problem, and these may lead the investigator to make a guess or formulate an hypothesis on it. Testing the hunch or hypothesis is the essential ingredient of an analytical study.

Types of Analytical Studies

Suppose that a descriptive study of chronic bronchitis in a suburban industrial area revealed a high rate of the disease among the entire population. While it may appear "obvious" that the "cause" of this problem is the air pollution produced by the local industries, there may be other causes of the problem. It is necessary, therefore, to test the hypothesis more specifically by conducting analytical studies on the specific population. The following are typical examples of the kinds of studies that could be designed for this purpose.

1. Compare the rate of chronic bronchitis for those people residing immediately adjacent to the industrial plants to that for residents living in the surrounding area.

2. Compare the rate of chronic bronchitis in the research population to that in another, nonindustrial community with similar demographic characteristics, a "twin community."

3. Select two groups of teenagers who do not have chronic bronchitis, one group from the target community and the other group from a nonindustrial community. Compare the development of chronic bronchitis in the two groups over a span of years.

4. By testing the amount of particulate matter in the area, determine residential areas that are high, medium, and low in pollution density. Compare rates and development of chronic bronchitis in the three areas over a span of years.

5. Since smoking and overcrowding are known to be related to chronic bronchitis, determine the occurrence of the disease among nonsmokers and those living in noncrowded conditions.

Each of these studies is purposely designed to accumulate data that can be used to test a predetermined hypothesis: air pollution is causally related to chronic bronchitis. It is important to note, however, that such studies do not *prove* a causal relationship, but they do add significant strength to the hypothesis that such a relationship does or does not exist.

As supportive data accumulate among more population groups with consistent results over a period of time, the likelihood of a true causal relationship becomes greater. Although this remains in the realm of judgment rather than proof, it is often sufficient to justify preventive action or treatment. As mentioned earlier, a prime example is the antismoking campaigns which resulted primarily from a massive accumulation of circumstantial evidence linking lung cancer with cigarette smoking which was gathered from descriptive and analytical studies.

Prospective Studies. If an epidemiologist wished to study the relationship between asbestos "dust" and lung cancer, he would most likely conduct a *prospective study*. This study would involve the selection of a population sample composed of new employees in asbestos factories who have not yet been exposed to the suspected hazardous substance. The subjects would then be monitored for a number of years to determine the extent to which they contracted lung cancer. If the rate of lung cancer cases in this group is significantly higher than that in the general population, then it can be concluded that a probable relationship between asbestos dust and lung cancer does exist. If additional studies of asbestos workers reveal similar results, some form of preventive action is warranted, even though a direct cause-and-effect relationship has not been established.

A prospective study is the selection and follow-up over a span of years of a sample population which has or has not been exposed to suspected disease-producing conditions. The extent to which disease occurs in the group after a certain amount of time is then compared to the "average" or existing rate of occurrence in the general population. From these comparisons, conclusions can be drawn as to the probable relationship between the exposure factor and the development of the disease.

Retrospective Studies. When samples of population groups are studied by analyzing or checking records of past experience with or exposure to suspected causative substances, a *retrospective study* is being conducted. The subjects sampled in most retrospective studies have the specific disease condition(s) being studied. The investigator looks for some common element in the past histories of the patients that might bear on their disease condition or tries to determine past exposure to hypothesized causes. Such studies can be accomplished more efficiently and quickly than prospective studies, but often they suffer from having to rely on the memory of the patients. Objective records of the past, such as hospital records, are much more desirable sources of such information.

Cohort and case-control techniques. Both prospective and retrospective studies commonly employ special techniques designed to reduce the sources of error or of bias and to increase the validity of the conclusions reached. *Cohort studies* use a sample group that does not have the disease being studied or that has not been exposed to the suspected cause of the disease. In the asbestos dust example, the investigator would study a second sample group of persons who are drawn from the same residential population as the factory workers but who are not factory employees. This group would be monitored for an equal number of years, and its rate of lung cancer would be compared statistically to that of the factory workers. In a retrospective study, the cohort group would consist of people who did not have the disease in question. Their past experiences or records would be evaluated for exposure to a suspected causative factor and compared to the case group.

In all uses of the cohort technique, a crucial element is the sample source of both groups. The populations from which they are drawn must be similar. If the case group is composed of hospital patients, then the cohort group should also be hospital patients. If the case group is made up of sixth graders from a rural school, then the cohort group should be sixth graders from another rual school with similar characteristics.

The cohort technique is taken one step further in the *case-control method.* This technique requires the selection of a control, or cohort, group in which each subject is "matched" with a subject in the case group. In other words, each cohort subject would be identical to a case subject in such characteristics as age, sex, marital status, educational level, and socioeconomic status. The similarity of the two groups provides some control of variables that might otherwise be a source of bias in the study. This control provides greater reliability in the total conduct of the study and substantially increases the validity of the conclusions. When done well, a case-control study is a close approximation of the experimental method discussed in the following section.

EXPERIMENTAL STUDIES

The application of specific research principles in the search for cause-and-effect relationships is fundamental to any science. To determine indisputably the specific cause or causes of a particular occurrence is the primary purpose of experimental epidemiology. The epidemiologist's ability to draw definite conclusions from his research depends on his strict adherence to the following basic research principles.

1. *Control of variables.* Theoretically, all factors that could conceivably affect the experimental results should be under the control of the researcher. If the carcinogenic effects of coal tar on the skin of experimental animals are being studied, then the genetic characteristics of the animals should be similar, diets should be the same, environmental conditions equal, dosage rates and times precisely the same, and so forth. If all other variables which could potentially influence the results are under control, then

the researcher can conclude that any skin changes are the result of the application of coal tar.

2. *Randomization.* To ensure that experimental groups are similar in all respects prior to the research treatment, subjects are randomly assigned to research groups in such a way that all members of the original population have an equal chance of being placed in any group. In the coal tar experiment, a lottery system or table of random numbers could be used to place the rats into the desired number of groups.

3. *Control treatment.* A control group is necessary to provide a means of comparing the results of treatment versus nontreatment. A control group is similar in all respects to the research group with the exception of the experimental treatment. For example, one group of rats in the coal tar experiment would not receive the coal tar application or would receive skin applications of an inert substance.

4. *Blindness.* It is usually undesirable for the experimenter to know which group is being treated and which is not. Therefore, in a blind experiment he is unaware, for exam-

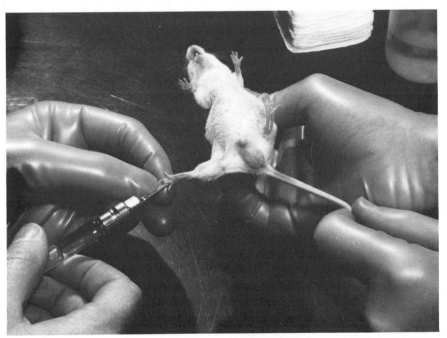

Laboratory animals are often used in experimental studies. *(Center for Disease Control, U.S. Public Health Service)*

ple, which rats are being treated with coal tar and which are receiving applications of an inert substance. If two subject groups are monitored, it is called a "double blind" experiment; if three groups are used, it is termed a "triple blind" technique. The purpose of this procedure is to eliminate any bias or favoritism on the part of the experimenter.

The conditions required for experimental studies restrict their application primarily to laboratory situations where complete control is possible. On occasion, however, experimental studies have been conducted in the field, but in most instances the factors involved in the studies have been highly specific, such as the effectiveness of a specific therapeutic agent or vaccine. There are also instances in the literature of experimentation in which humans have been exposed to suspected causative agents in attempts to produce the disease. Such experiments, however, are strongly attacked on

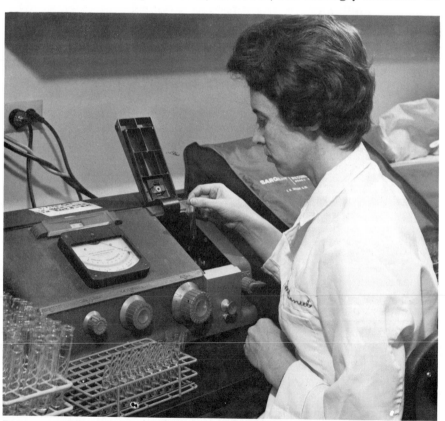

Because complete control is required in experimental studies, they are usually **carried out** in the laboratory. *(Center for Disease Control, U.S. Public Health Service)*

moral grounds and are not commonly conducted in modern research programs.

Experimental studies cannot be fully successful in the community setting because they cannot fully control the emotional, social, and pyschological characteristics of their human subjects. While such studies may be designed according to experimental principles and even be called experimental, their conclusions will always be less than definitive because of the presence of these changeable factors in human nature.

The question of causation in epidemiology is a crucial one. Rarely is the investigator of community health problems provided the luxury of conditions so neatly controlled that one single cause can be clearly isolated. (Incidents of food poisoning and isolated outbreaks of specific infectious diseases are common exceptions, however.) Statistical manipulations can never be considered as proof of "cause"; all they can do is give supportive evidence to suspicions of a cause. As A. R. Feinstein states, "The general issue of how to prove cause is neither clinical nor statistical; it is a matter of logic and what constitutes a valid form of reasoning with statistics."[1] In the face of health problems that defy laboratory experimentation and precision, the value of descriptive and analytical studies and the validity of their design and interpretations cannot be underestimated.

SOURCES OF EPIDEMIOLOGICAL DATA

All epidemiological studies require the collection and analysis of data derived from population groups. Such data comprise the raw materials from which descriptive pictures of population groups and health problems are completed, from which hypotheses are generated and tested, and upon which the conclusions of experimental research are based. A vast network of standardized data-collection procedures is available to epidemiologists for these studies, and specific techniques for "customized" or localized collection of information continue to be developed.

Standardized procedures refer to the predetermined methods for the collection and central accumulation of data on a national scope. The data collected and the procedures used are established and regulated by law. *Localized procedures,* on the other hand, are applied to specific population groups for the study of specific health problems. Data are collected and analyses made by epidemiologists in response to felt needs, generally as they occur, on the local level.

STANDARDIZED SOURCES OF DATA

The need for compiling statistical records of the population of this country was recognized as early as the middle of the seventeenth century. Following English tradition, colonists mandated the recording of marriages, christenings, and burials for the primary purpose of protecting individual rights, especially with respect to the ownership and distribution of property. Little thought was given to the use of such records for health purposes, but in effect they provided a documented account of births, marriages, and deaths as they occurred among specified population groups. However primitive and sporadic these early records may have been, they were firmly established on the principle that such records are legal statements of fact, existing primarily for the administration of justice and the protection of individual rights. The systematic use of such records for health purposes was not to come for two centuries, by which time the methods and procedures of data collection were well rehearsed.

Census Data

The United States Constitution decrees that beginning in 1790 and for every 10 years thereafter a complete enumeration, or *census,* of the population be taken. The original purpose of the census was to determine the number of members of the House of Representatives each state was entitled to according to its population. Over the years, however, additional items have been added to the census questionnaire so that current census data include significant information on the demography of the United States population. On national, state, county and city bases, population "mixes" according to such factors as sex, age, race, residence, and education can be determined and compared from decade to decade. The kind of information gathered in the census that would be of particular interest to the epidemiologist includes:

    I. General and social characteristics
1. Race
2. Date and place of birth
3. Years of school completed by age, occupation, income, and poverty status
4. Marital status and marital history
5. Families by type and composition, income, and poverty status
6. Fertility
7. Work disability
8. Residence

II. Economic characteristics
1. Employment status
2. Occupation
3. Income
4. Poverty status

The value of census data to the community health profession is enormous. Population trends can be monitored to assist in the early prediction of developing health problems and to plan services and programs to meet impending needs. The rural to urban migration, the increase of women in the work force, the declining proportion of males to females, the sharp increase in the elderly population, the urban centralization of low-income families—all are trends systematically documented by census data, and each represents an area of special concern to the community health profession.

Census data have become so important to government, business, and social, educational, as well as health planners that procedures have been established by the census bureau to collect similar information during inter-census years. Current population surveys, using scientifically selected population samples from 357 areas of the United States, are conducted on a monthly basis. Based on statistical analyses of the samples, future population levels are projected for birth and death rates and net immigration and migration figures.

Through census procedures and interim population reports, a constant flow of population data is available to the community health worker which makes possible not only the projection of trends and future program needs on national and state levels, but also a statistical picture, or demographic "profile," of nearly every population group in the United States. While all communities have certain health needs and problems in common, each community experiences some special difficulties that are often the product of its particular population "mix." The community health worker would be well advised to plot systematically the demographic profile of his community and to maintain a constant source of data input to chart the flow of change in the population characteristics.

Vital Statistics

Population data are of significant value for planning and prediction purposes. Moreover, their value is increased when combined with information pertinent to specific health-related events. These combinations of health (or disease) data with population data are referred to as *vital statistics* and are presented in the form of rates as outlined in Table 6.1.

The law in all states requires that certain events related to health and disease be systematically registered and permanently recorded at the federal level. These events are birth, death, disease, marriage, and divorce. As the major events in human life they are called vital events, and the vital statistics are based on them.

Over 7,500,000 cases of birth, death, marriage, and divorce were registered in 1970. Many agencies and citizens used these records for a myriad of personal, legal, and health reasons. Vital statistics are essential to the planning and operation of health programs, education, social welfare, business enterprises, and a wide variety of other activities that pertain to the well-being of the population. Though still the most important users, the health and medical professions represent only one segment of the population that benefits from access to vital statistics.

The major function of vital statistics is to chart as accurately as possible the occurrence of vital events as they appear in the population as a whole and in specific population groups. The sample data in Figure 6.1 indicate some of the ways this information is presented. Such presentations have significant applications in the fields of medicine and community health; no other source of data can provide the continuous, past-to-present panoramic view of the current status and emerging trends of the health of the nation.

Registration of Vital Events: Births and Deaths. Procedures for the reporting of births and deaths are determined by law in each state. Local registrars are charged with receiving proper documen-

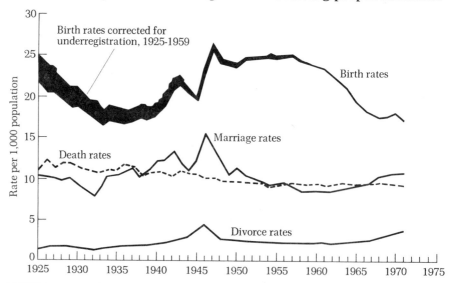

FIGURE 6.1. Vital statistics rates: United States, 1925–1971. *(Chart prepared by U.S. Bureau of the Census. Data from U.S. Public Health Service)*

tation from physicians and funeral directors, issuing the appropriate certificates, and forwarding the documents on to the proper health authorities at the state level. Although procedures vary somewhat, the certificates are then sent to the National Center for Health Statistics in Washington where the data are permanently recorded, analyzed, and published annually in *Vital Statistics of the United States.* Reporting of vital statistics from local to national level is shown in Figure 6.2.

Mortality data provide information not only on the number of deaths but also on the primary causes of death. By this means, shifts in major disease problems can be identified as they occur. As we have often noted, there have been dramatic changes in the leading causes of death in the United States during the first half of this century (see Table 2.1).

In addition to making available crude mortality data, death registration also provides the information from which mortality and death causation can be analyzed demographically. A death certificate not only fulfills the legal requirement for death registration but also records pertinent characteristics of the deceased such as age, sex, and education (see Figure 6.3). From this information such rates as infant mortality, age-specific, race-specific, and sex-specific mortality in any residential segment of the population can be computed and compared.

The law in all states requires that every live birth be recorded, certified, and reported following procedures similar to that of death registration. Documentation of birth is completed by the attending physician on a certificate of live birth (Figure 6.4). In addition to information legally required for certification, demographic and personal information about the parents is also included. Although personal medical facts may be kept confidential, facts recorded about conditions of pregnancy and childbirth, legitimacy, prematurity, congenital defects, and so on, provide vital information for research, treatment, and prevention of problems related to pregnancy.

Reporting of Notifiable Disease. The incidence of disease is included among the vital events, and thus must be reported according to the legal procedures described in Figure 6.2. While notification procedures are similar in all states, the number and kind of diseases which must be reported vary considerably. In most states, weekly reports similar to that shown in Table 6.2 are published. On the national level, the Center for Disease Control (formerly the National Communicable Disease Center) of the Public Health Service publishes a weekly list of 25 notifiable diseases in its *Mortality and Morbidity* reports.

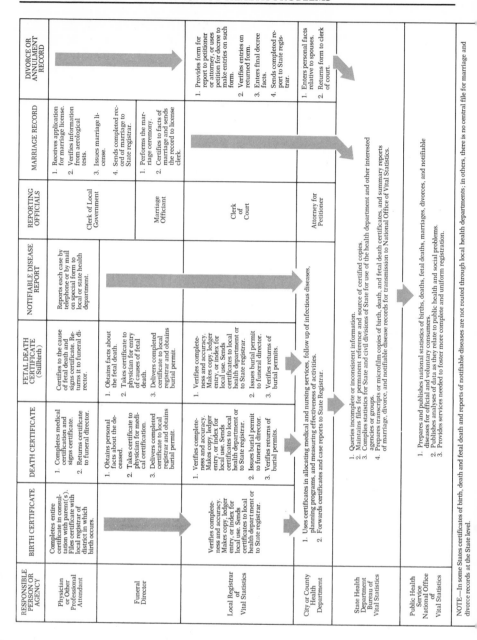

FIGURE 6.2.   Flow of vital record and statistics in the United States. (Vital Statistics of the United States, *Vol. I, 1950*)

Morbidity Statistics.   Morbidity is the amount of illness in a population. In most instances, it is measured for a particular disease in a particular population, such as the occurrence of lung cancer among men. Morbidity measurements may be of a more general nature, however, in which case a population is studied to determine the incidence of all diseases existing in it. Sources of morbidity data vary widely and include reports of notifiable diseases, health surveys, screening programs, and medical examinations of special population groups such as school children, pregnant women, and the aged. Morbidity statistics are the primary measurements used for assessing the relative importance or severity of a given health problem at a given time or over an extended period of time. Also, by providing data by which the scope and importance of various health problems can be compared, they are a valuable source of information that is used in determining priorities in health programming.

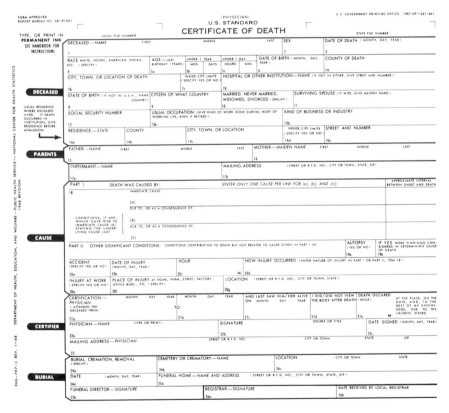

FIGURE 6.3.   Certificate of death. *(National Center for Health Statistics, U.S. Public Health Service)*

The computation of morbidity statistics is similar to the procedure discussed earlier in this chapter. There is one principal difference, however, that is important in the meaningful interpretation of the data and its value as a public health tool. In calculating morbidity rates, the population used in the denominator is often the number of people who are susceptible to the disease in question. This group is called the *population at risk.* Examples of health problems that have fairly well defined populations at risk are complications of pregnancy (pregnant women) and acute leukemia (children ages 2 to 15). The formula for computing infant mortality, as seen in Table 6.1, uses the number of live births in the denominator because they are the exclusive population to which the vital event can occur. (For diseases in which the total population is at risk, such as influenza, the at-risk rate would be the same as the crude rate.) At-risk morbidity statistics provide a more accurate measurement of the scope, intensity, and changing natures of certain health problems because they are not affected by changes in the numbers and composition of the entire population and because

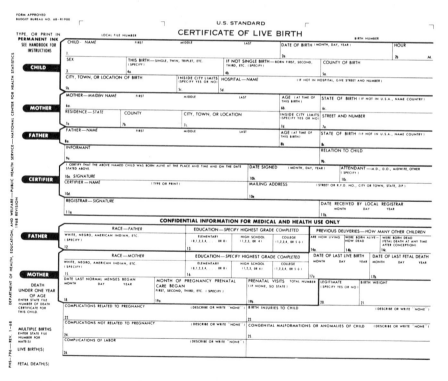

FIGURE 6.4.   Certificate of live birth. *(National Center for Health Statistics, U.S. Public Health Service)*

TABLE 6.2 Weekly report: Division of Disease Control, Illinois Department of Public Health. Provisional case reports, week ending June 21, 1974*

Disease	State totals				Cumulative totals to date			
					State		Chicago	
	This week 1974	Same week 1973	Last week 1974	Five year median	1974	1974	1974	1973
Chickenpox	184	273	202	109	6,222	11,935	513	684
Diphtheria	0	0	0	0	2	0	2	0
Encephalitis, acute	0	1	1		5	23	4	9
Gonorrhea	1,016	526	622		21,098	20,244	14,160	13,796
Hepatitis A & Unspec	53	67	35		1,016	986	311	321
Hepatitis B	9	17	9		201	145	86	38
Measles	33	67	94	67	1,573	1,790	457	820
Meningitis:								
Meningococcic	0	2	0		11	31	5	7
Other bacterial	6	10	7		90	123	39	48
Aseptic	0	2	0		12	24	4	2
Mumps	53	55	36		999	2,309	228	243
Poliomyelitis	0	0	0	0	1	0	0	0
Rabies:								
Heads examined	124	166	158		2,315	2,716	239	264
Positive heads	3	4	4		62	159	0	0
Treatments	6	0	0		34	83	0	14
Rheumatic Fever	2	7	3		65	444	45	66
Rubella	4	45	8		372	1,037	25	41
Scarlet Fever	5	12	40	8	724	625	78	64
Syphilis:								
Primary & secondary	14	2	9		595	96	468	—
Total	42	74	102		2,752	2,123	2,111	1,320
Tuberculosis	31	44	23		711	695	503	500
Typhoid Fever	0	1	0	0	5	9	4	5
Whooping Cough	4	1	2	1	121	36	103	15

* From the Illinois State Department of Public Health

the groups involved are more precisely defined and objectively measurable.

To strengthen the value and usefulness of morbidity data, two measures of morbidity are commonly used; *incidence rates* and *prevalence rates.* The incidence rate for a health problem is computed by the number of *new cases* that occur during a given period of time, divided by the number of persons in the at-risk population, multiplied by 1,000 or 100,000. Incidence statistics allow the continual monitoring of immediately developing trends in disease occurrence.

Prevalence rates are based on the number of cases of a disease which exist at a given time, regardless of their time of origin, within a given population. These rates are used primarily to describe the existing status and severity of health problems and in assessing trends as they develop over extended periods of time.

The Question of Accuracy

An awesome amount of data is gathered through the legal procedures for the collection and recording of vital statistics, and a great deal of care must be exercised in interpreting the data and in drawing inferences and conclusions from them. The system is far from perfect, and its deficiencies should be well known to the community health professional.

First, the recording procedures depend on the efficiency and accuracy with which vital events are reported by physicians, hospitals, and funeral directors. On occasion, medical personnel may not have sufficient information to diagnose diseases or to determine precise causes of death. In addition, some physicians and hospitals are reluctant to report the occurrence of some diseases, such as venereal disease or mental illnesses. Simple negligence is also a factor in failures to report vital events. Incomplete or faulty information introduces a source of bias that reduces the confidence with which the data can be meaningfully interpreted.

Secondly, generally uniform registration procedures were not established in all states until the mid-1930s. For this reason, comparisons of vital rates occurring before and after the 1930s present a somewhat distorted picture. In one Illinois rural town in 1878, for example, deaths were recorded for "ceretites," "abdominal acetes," and various "inflammations" of the lung, bowel, brain, and liver, but such data defy classification and comparison with those gathered on specific conditions causing death today.

A third imperfection in the vital statistics system is that the definitions of some vital events are not uniform across all states and among countries of the world. Fetal deaths, for example, are defined as "death prior to complete expulsion from its mother of a product of conception, regardless of the duration of pregnancy; the death is indicated by the fact that after such separations the fetus does not breathe or show any other evidence of life, such as beating of the heart, pulsation of the umbilical cord. . . . If a child breathes or shows any other evidence of life after complete birth, even though it be only momentary, the birth should be registered as a live birth and a death certificate also should be filed."[2]

Despite the reasonable clarity of the definition and the inclusion of the phrase "regardless of the duration of pregnancy," statistical confusion occurs because certain states and countries retain a minimal gestation period in their identification of fetal death. A gestation period of 20 weeks, for example, may be required for designation of a fetal death, with fetuses under 20 weeks being excluded from any form of registration. Moreover, according to the definition here of live birth, an infant born at any time during pregnancy which shows any evidence of life must be considered a live birth. If the infant dies, even within minutes after birth, both a birth and death certificate must be recorded.

Since there is no universal agreement on or interpretation of definitions of births and fetal deaths, statistics on these vital events should not be taken at face value, especially in the comparison of rates among countries. The use of different criteria for determining either of these vital events significantly affects not only the birth and fetal death statistics but also the infant mortality rate, since the calculations of this rate are made from both recorded births and deaths within the first years of life.

Despite its imperfections, the system of registration and compilation of vital statistics provides an invaluable source of data to nearly all segments of the health and social professions. Many national and local programs of treatment and prevention are structured on the basis of vital statistics, and these statistics are the most important single source of data upon which projections of future health problems and needs can be made. In sum, vital statistics constitute the most basic and reliable element in this country's system of health intelligence.

National Health Survey

Although the value of vital statistics is beyond question, there remains a great deal of health information not readily available from national registration systems. The decline in communicable disease problems and the corresponding increase in chronic and degenerative diseases made it apparent that little was known about the scope and intensity of the latter types of diseases among the population as a whole. The need for more information on these conditions led Congress in 1956 to pass the National Health Survey Act. The legislation called for a continuous health survey program which was "to provide data on the incidence of illness and accidental injuries; the prevalence of disease and impairment; the extent of disability; the volume and kinds of medical, dental, and hospital care received; and other health-related problems."[3]

Data for the NHS are collected from samples of a cross-section of the population; three different kinds of survey are used in gathering the data: (1) health interview survey, (2) health and nutrition examination survey, and (3) health records survey.

Health Interview Survey. A sample of approximately 40,000 households throughout the country are randomly selected for inclusion in this survey. Household interviews are conducted on a continuous basis, reaching about 700 households a week. While the topics

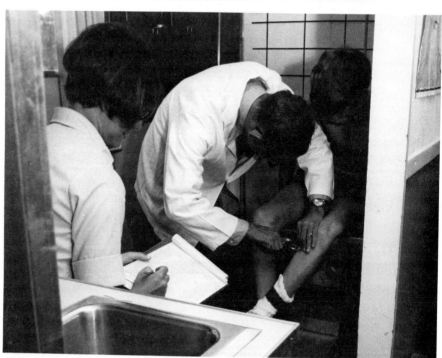

Body measurements are taken as a part of the Health and Nutrition Examination Survey. *(National Center for Health Statistics, U.S. Public Health Service)*

of the surveys vary from year to year, they are most commonly concerned with the occurrence and treatment of chronic diseases. An important by-product of this survey is the accumulation of information on the social and economic impact of chronic illness on both the patient and his family.

Health and Nutrition Examination Survey. Physical examinations and clinical tests form this survey's basis. Selected population samples are brought to mobile examination centers for evaluations of general physical health, blood pressure, and cholesterol levels, and for the possible discovery of evidence of chronic diseases and disabilities. Population samples are drawn from specific age groups in order to obtain more precise information on the age-related characteristics of chronic diseases.

Health Records Survey. This survey calls for the creation and maintenance of a central file of all health-related institutions in the United States. Hospitals, clinics, professional offices, nursing homes, and correctional institutions are among the major facilities cataloged. In addition, this survey collects information on the institutionalized segments of the population, with special emphasis on the chronically ill and disabled.

The National Health Survey and the Vital Registration System are the major sources of data collected on a nation-wide basis. They are not limited to national use, however, but are available in published form to any interested agencies or individuals. The United States Bureau of the Census and the National Center for Health Statistics (United States Public Health Statistics) are charged with the responsibility of publishing and disseminating the population figures and the health-related data that in combination produce the vital statistics of the United States.

"LOCALIZED" SOURCES OF DATA

Faced with health needs and problems peculiar to his state or community, the epidemiologist must rely on data and information often not available by standardized means. A major portion of his responsibilities lies with the development and application of methods and procedures of data collection specifically for his population. It is one thing to know the venereal disease rate in the United States, but quite another to determine the extent of the disease among the teenage population of a medium-sized suburb. To collect and evaluate data for the identification of specific health problems in limited populations is the primary function of "localized" procedures such as field epidemiology, health surveys, community self-studies, and screening tests. Once the facts are known and a need well established, few citizens and community officials will oppose the establishment or improvement of local health services.

Field Epidemiology

The sudden emergence of a health or disease problem, such as food poisoning or epidemics, calls for the immediate application by the epidemiologist of specialized field procedures, including intense investigation and the marshalling of medical specialists for clinical and laboratory studies. The investigatory procedure is usually a predetermined, step-by-step process, although of necessity it does not always conform to a rigid pattern. With time the overriding factor in emergencies, several components of a field study will be carried out simultaneously.

The first step is to identify the scope of the problem—to determine if an epidemic or serious outbreak actually exists. The criterion used is the determination of the occurrence of new cases of a disease beyond the usual expectation at a particular time among a certain population. This expectation will vary: one or two cases of typhoid fever may constitute an epidemic in the United States, while it may take 30 to 40 cases to be considered an epidemic in other parts of the world.

Secondly, the specific diagnosis of the disease must be verified. Verification depends on not only clinical and laboratory procedures but also the reliability of reporting sources such as physicians, laboratories, and health departments.

Thirdly, the groups of cases under study should be classified according to definite, probable, and suspected cases in a particular community or population group. These groups should then be analyzed according to demographic variables (sex, age, and so on), geographic variables (region, sanitary subdivision) and temporal variables (hours, days, weeks) in an attempt to isolate the source of the outbreak. The purpose of such analysis is to determine common exposures, experiences, or living conditions of those with the disease. Practices in common, such as eating at the same restaurant, drinking from the same water supply, and exposure to the same carriers of an infectious disease, are important clues in determining the source and mode of transmission of the disease.

The fourth step is to establish and test an hypothesis on the type of epidemic, its sources, means of transmission, and so forth. Finally, conclusions are drawn and recommendations made for the control of the outbreak, treatment and care of cases, and the prevention of future outbreaks.

Health Surveys

The use of survey questionnaires and household interviews for collecting health data has been commonplace in community health practice since the advent of social and chronic health problems. Because sociological factors influence these problems significantly, the community health worker must be aware of the social as well as physical characteristics of his community as they pertain to its health. Health surveys of community populations are often conducted not only to determine the existence of specific disease problems but to assess such factors as utilization of health services, public knowledge and attitude toward health problems and pro-

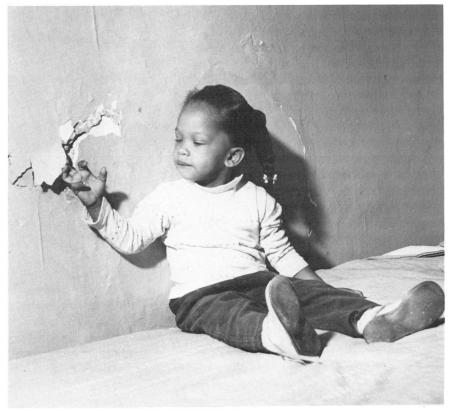

Health surveys were able to account for the increasing incidence of lead poisoning among inner-city children by demonstrating that the above-average level of lead in their blood resulted from a common practice among many of eating paint peeling off the walls. *(Courtesy of the American National Red Cross)*

grams, and social-psychological factors that may be affecting health behavior. The accumulated data allow the health professional to draw a more complete "health profile" of the community and to plan services and programs more effectively than would be possible from the assessment of physical health conditions alone.

In addition to broad-scope surveys to evaluate general health conditions and facilities, surveys are also designed to establish the existence of specific health needs and problems. A high incidence of specific types of disease in a local population may provoke such a survey. For example, one team of researchers surveyed a Puerto Rican community to determine the extent of mortality, morbidity, and decreased debility from water-borne diseases. Their purpose was to assess the value of modernizing the population's water supply system. An increased number of children living in inner-city housing have been hospitalized in recent years for lead poisoning. Blood tests of samples drawn from such populations in several major cities revealed that a large number of children had above-average lead content in their blood. Follow-up surveys verified that the condition was the result of the ingestion of paint peeling off the walls and that this practice was common among ghetto children. In economically depressed areas such as Appalachia, nutritional studies are commonly conducted to identify the specific dietary deficiencies that might account for high susceptibility to infectious diseases and the below-normal growth and maturation rates of the children of these areas.

Community Self-Studies

One of the contemporary trends in the community health field is the active involvement of the consumer in the planning, implementation, and operation of health programs. A part of this movement is the practice of community self-study: the gathering of data concerning health problems of the community and the effectiveness of existing programs and services in meeting the health needs of the population. Community self-studies are conducted for the purpose of taking inventories of health services as they exist in the community, identifying present needs for health services, and suggesting means to establish the services. Surveys of existing programs and services are conducted, along with interviews of community citizens to determine their views of local health problems and the extent to which they are willing to get involved in planning and implementing the needed services. Following the collection of data, plans for implementation are drawn and methods of converting plans into action are determined.

Under the sponsorship of the National Commission on Community Health Services, 21 community self-studies were conducted throughout the country during the 1960s. As seen by the following list of partial achievements, the results of this project clearly demonstrate its value.

1. Laws and practices for admitting the mentally ill to institutional care were changed;
2. Hospital and allied facilities were expanded along with the development of medical residency and medical research programs;
3. A 15,000,000 dollar bond issue was proposed to finance development of a medical complex. Over half of the revenue was to be spent for outpatient services, extended care facilities and other programs designed to meet the needs created by contemporary disease problems.
4. Three communities began developing areawide health departments.
5. An environmental health rural renewal league was formed, giving priority to housing, water supplies, and waste disposal.
6. Study recommendations related to a school health program were implemented by the state superintendent of Public Instruction.[4]

The basic unit of the community self-study is the action-planning group—a cross-section of the local citizenry forming a partnership among private, voluntary, professional, and governmental sectors of the community. The community health specialist is one of the most important members of the planning group. By working in a coordinated effort with other concerned citizens and professionals, he is afforded a vehicle by which his professional goals can be reached while at the same time he is able to establish firm relationships and lines of communication with all segments of the community. The community self-study not only is an informational tool of the health professional, but it also creates an organizational system through which continuous efforts at community health improvement may be channeled.

Screening Tests

Medical authorities recognize that although primary prevention of disease is the ultimate goal of the health profession, the complexity of today's socially related diseases make such a goal at present unattainable. However, secondary prevention—halting the progress of a disease from its early, often undetected stage to a more severe one—is becoming more of a reality because of the improved efficiency and effectiveness of *screening tests.* These tests involve the application of specific medical and laboratory techniques designed to identify possible or probable disease conditions. They are intended not as final diagnosis but for the identification of persons who should be referred to physicians for more complete examinations.

The most complete form of secondary prevention is the annual health examination, including medical history, complete medical examination, laboratory tests, guidance, and follow-up. However, such examinations cannot be completely successful among population groups because of the limitations of time, cost, facilities, and the inherent difficulties in diagnosing some disease conditions.

In an attempt to counteract some of these deficiencies, the practice of multiphasic screening has evolved. A number of disease conditions can be tested by a variety of screening techniques: diabetes, anemia, and venereal disease from one blood sample; tuberculosis, lung cancer, and heart defects from the same chest X ray; diabetes and kidney disorders from a urine sample. This procedure has the definite advantages of being fast, inexpensive, convenient to the consumer, and readily conducted by nonmedical personnel. In addition, the benefits of early detection can be brought conveniently to large population groups such as hospital patients, industrial and

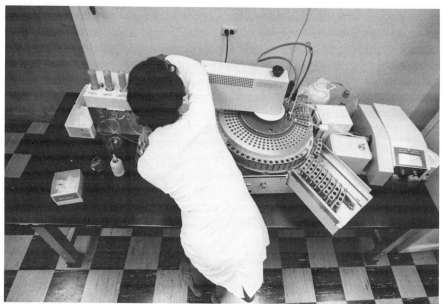

Automated laboratory equipment for the analysis of fats, sugar, and protein in the blood helps make mass examinations possible. *(Courtesy of the World Health Organization)*

labor groups, residents of nursing homes, and students. Group data such as these are of great potential value to the community health specialists and program planners as well as to the group members themselves.

SUMMARY

One of the basic responsibilities of the epidemiologist is to gather and analyze specific data about a community health problem in order to contribute to the development of control measures. Three specific types of studies are conducted for this purpose. *Descriptive studies* are designed to gather and categorize data in such a way that a given population, usually composed of people with a specific health problem or exhibiting specific health-related behavior, can be identified demographically. The purpose of the study is to identify common characteristics of the population that might assist in further understanding of the health problem under investigation. Descriptive data are usually converted into rates in order for comparisons of population groups to be made.

In many instances, descriptive studies will suggest hypotheses for further investigation by the epidemiologist. *Analytical studies* are designed to test these hypotheses. While such studies do not prove a causal relationship, they do provide evidence as to the validity of the hypothesized relationship. Prospective and retrospective studies are the most common kinds of analytical investigations conducted.

Experimental studies are designed specifically to test an hypothesized cause-and-effect relationship. Since specific principles of research design must be followed strictly, most experimental studies are carried out under laboratory conditions. Firm cause-and-effect conclusions are rarely justified in studies conducted out in the field, even though the basic principles of experimental research design are followed.

The data used in epidemiological investigations are collected in many ways from a large number of sources. Standardized procedures for data collection are composed of a broad network of informational sources which are national in scope and regulated by law. Census data and vital statistics are the most commonly used sources of standardized health data. Localized sources of data are those used by the epidemiologist to study specific population groups and health problems peculiar to his state or community. Field studies, local health surveys, and community self-studies are the typical procedures for the collection of localized data.

REFERENCES

1. A. R. Feinstein, *Clinical Judgement* (Baltimore: Williams and Wilkins Co., 1967), p. 62.
2. National Office of Vital Statistics, *Physician's Handbook on Death and Birth Registration,* 11th ed., Public Health Service, 1958, p. 15.
3. National Center for Health Statistics, *Origin, Program and Operation of the U.S. National Health Survey,* Public Health Service Publication 1000, Series 1, No. 1, 1963, p. 8.
4. National Commission on Community Health Services, *Health Is a Community Affair* (Cambridge, Mass.: Harvard University Press, 1966) p. 230.

TOPICS FOR DISCUSSION

1. Select a specific health problem, such as smoking and lung cancer or diet and heart disease, and prepare in outline form designs for descriptive, analytical, and experimental studies related to that problem.
2. Discuss the kinds of conclusions that can be justified in the conducting of descriptive, analytical, and experimental studies. In what instances would an epidemiologist be justified in making program decisions based on the data from these types of studies?
3. Why are crude rates of only limited value in the description and analysis of health data? What other types of rates could be used to produce more reliable descriptions or comparisons of population groups?
4. Suppose a health agency in your community were to apply for a grant to establish a well-baby clinic. How might that agency utilize both standardized and localized data-collection procedures in order to gather the information necessary to justify the request?

Part Three

Meeting Community Health Needs

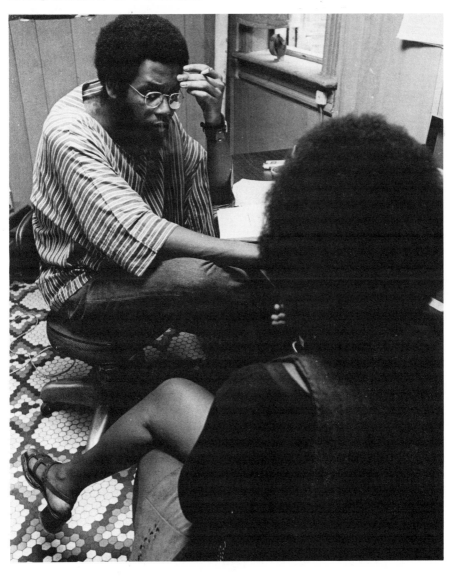

In his interview with a woman considering taking up residence in a local drug-rehabilitation center, the drug counselor tries to assess her interest in and commitment to the program. *(Photo on previous page courtesy of the World Health Organization)*

7. Organization for Community Health

The concept of the whole individual functioning effectively in his environment has come to represent the ideal of health. In working from this perspective, however, it is often difficult to differentiate between what is health related and what is not. Consequently, the designation of a health-related organization or activity becomes nebulous when many necessary health activities are being performed by groups or organizations not usually considered part of the health field. For example, a local ladies club may operate a nutrition program for the elderly in a community, or a fraternal group such as the Eagles may provide hospital beds for patients at home. Similarly, welfare organizations, drug companies, philanthropic foundations, and professional associations provide some input into the total community health field. Thus, this broad, comprehensive view of health leads to a diversity of activities and groups operable under such a definition. It also makes a clear dichotomy between health and nonhealth groups extemely difficult.

Nonetheless, it is useful to devise a framework from which to study the organization for community health. This model involves a review both of the functions performed within the health system and of the organizations and individuals who perform them. The first part of the model has been developed by Mary F. Arnold and is based on the thesis that the health system, encompassing the whole repertoire of community health activities, serves two needs of society: "maintenance of a positive biological relationship to the environment and prevention of disruptive behaviors attributed by the society to ill health."[1] The second part of the model divides the organizations into various groupings in order to aid in assessing their importance and their contributions. In each instance the major functions of the group will be placed within the previous functional perspective.

THE FUNCTIONAL MODEL OF HEALTH-RELATED ACTIVITIES

Any distinctions concerning the basic functions within a total health system have to be somewhat arbitrary. But if we start with the original premise that the health system serves two societal needs—maintenance and prevention—then it is possible to develop four broad categories of activities that seek to meet these needs. Figure 7.1 presents the four groups of activities and the support elements necessary for the operation of these activities. A closer look at each of these four activities will provide a salient perspective for understanding the place and importance of the agencies, institutions, and individuals within the community health field.

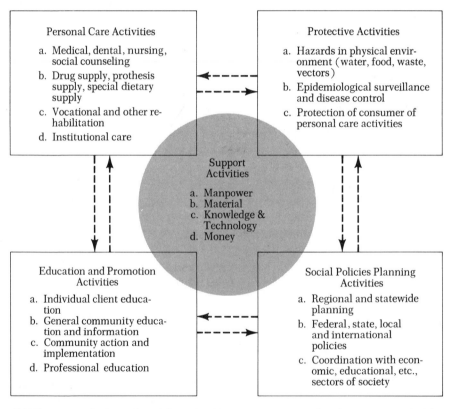

FIGURE 7.1.   A functional model of a health system. *(Reprinted with permission of Aldine Atherton, Inc., publisher)*

Personal Care Activities

Personal care activities include the cure and treatment of health problems and, more recently, preventive measures such as yearly medical exams, pap smears, immunizations, and a variety of diagnostic tests and examinations. A labyrinth of individuals and organizations is involved in these activities, including hospitals, clinics, nursing homes, counseling groups, rehabilitation services, and such professionals as doctors, nurses, dentists, therapists, and medical technicians.

It is this group of activities that is most identified in the layman's mind with the concept of health—an association rooted in society's emphasis on the cure and treatment of health problems rather than on their prevention. Such activities represent the direct services that are desired when one is ill. Because of the immediacy and magnitude of the need, these services have historically been given priority in the development of the health system. Only recently has preventive medicine become an important feature of direct service activities, and it still runs a distant second to the curative aspect.

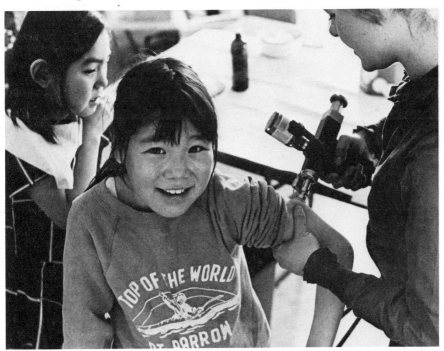

Personal Care Activities. Immunization against communicable diseases is one of the measures most often associated by the public with health care. *(Center for Disease Control, U.S. Public Health Service)*

Though this broad functional area commands the greatest amount of input in relation to manpower, material, and knowledge, we will see that the other three areas are gaining in importance and seem to presage a greater concern for health maintenance rather than repair.

Protective Activities

With increasing knowledge concerning the causes of disease and illness there has been a concomitant development of activities designed to protect against exposure to those causative elements. As discussed in Chapter 6, epidemiology has provided a scientific method to determine cause-and-effect relationships and has given rise to a host of concepts regarding protection against health problems. Witness, for example, the number of regulations and stand-

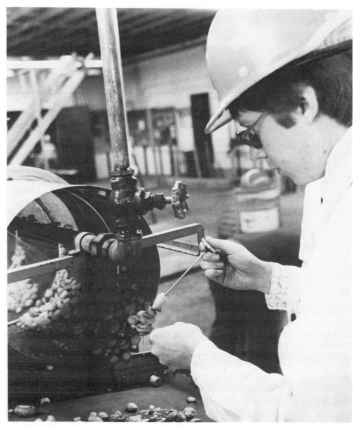

Protective Activities. A consumer safety officer checks mushroom temperature after the blanching operation, during which the product is heated. *(Food and Drug Administration, U.S. Public Health Service)*

ards concerning water supplies, food handling, air pollution, and waste disposal. The great advances in immunization and the programs in rodent and insect control can be traced back to our understandings of cause and effect.

But these are only a few of the protective activities. In industry, occupational safety is a major health concern, and much effort has been aimed at providing safe working conditions. Recently there has been a good deal of emphasis on consumer protection, with concern voiced over unsafe products and false, misleading advertising. At both the national and state levels, the Environmental Protection Agency has emerged as a powerful force, figuring prominently in such controversies as strip-mining legislation and the Alaskan pipeline. Further, the "Naderism" voice has buttressed the activities of the government's Consumer Protection Agency whose role has continually grown in response to continuing consumer awareness and consequent demands.

This group of activities will most likely become more and more important in view of the increasing emphasis on environmental problems, on greater government involvement in health matters, and on prevention rather than cure. The environmental issue has already resulted in antipollution regulations, greater regulation in food packaging, and closer scrutiny of all technological developments with possible detrimental effects on health. The government has become a major force in this whole realm of protection and is largely responsible for the proliferation of protective activities throughout the nation, which are based on the underlying theme of prevention as opposed to cure.

Education and Promotion Activities

An enlightened and willing public is a necessary component of an effective health system. The effectiveness of even the most elaborate program can be measured only as a function of the number of people that are aided by it or the number of problems it can alleviate. Consequently, the education of the public and the promotion of the health program are as important as the health program itself. This is especially true in view of contemporary health problems where individual motivation is the prime factor determining participation in health programs.

Much to the dismay of health professionals, it has often been found that well-intentioned services or programs were totally avoided by the target population because of misunderstanding, fear, or a variety of socio-cultural intangibles. Recognition of this fact has led to current emphasis on public health education and more in-

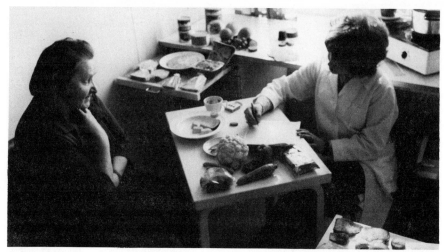

Health Education. A dietician explains nutrition and prepares a diet-sheet for a patient to enable her to maintain a suitable and healthful diet outside the health center. *(Courtesy of the World Health Organization)*

volvement of the consumer in actual program planning. This emphasis on the consumer has, in most cases, aided the promotion of programs in communities where public distrust has hindered health programs in the past.

In addition to concern for the public in general, attention has been increasingly focused on health education in schools and on the individual in personal counseling sessions. Many states have passed legislation requiring health education courses to be taught at both the junior and senior high school levels.

Realizing the importance of education and promotion, community health leaders have, in recent times, increased their efforts in educational and promotional programs, and most health agencies now employ at least one full-time person in health education. In addition, many voluntary health agencies exist almost solely to educate the public on health matters. Programs to prepare health education specialists are burgeoning in colleges around the country. In the succeeding sections of this chapter the magnitude of the education and promotion activities will become even more apparent.

Social Policies Planning Activities

Planning has become a pervasive term in the rhetoric of community work. Given the pluralism of social needs and the maze of public and private agencies to meet these needs, inadequate planning can result in poor coordination, needless duplication, and costly waste of both personnel and materials. This is certainly true within the health system.

As already mentioned, the government has greatly increased its involvement in the health field. Programs in mental health, family planning, nutrition, and for the aged have been initiated at local levels through state coordinating agencies backed by federal funding. There are community public health departments, welfare organizations, rehabilitation services, and a conglomerate of public agencies directly or indirectly involved in health-related activities. Juxtapose these government facilities with the number of voluntary agencies (such as the American Cancer Society and the National Heart Association), professional groups (such as the American Medical Association), and philanthropic foundations that are involved in health-related programs, and the need for planning and coordination becomes obvious.

With so many groups interested and active in the health field it is possible to find two or more organizations attacking the same problem, overlapping in services and programs, and deriving no benefit from the existence of each other. Effective planning could decrease this overlap, allow for profitable exchange between agencies, and increase the range of services as well as the number of problems actively pursued.

Support Activities

The maintenance of these four categories of activities requires support activities. For example, the health manpower needs alone are tremendous. Besides the obviously necessary health personnel such as doctors, nurses, and technicians, there are educators, administrators, planners, and various ancillary personnel which are all vital to the system. Add to the manpower requirements all the activities necessary to raise money, supply material, and develop technology, and the number of support activities appears awesome.

At this point, no attempt will be made to discuss separately each of these activities. It should be possible, however, to infer their importance as we move through the organizational framework in the following pages. Suffice it to say that the support activities are the basic fuels that run the complex health machine.

HEALTH-RELATED ORGANIZATIONS

Having discussed the functional model, we may now turn to the complex organizational framework through which these activities

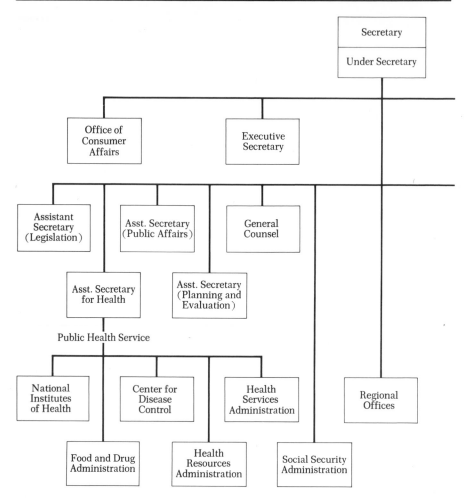

FIGURE 7.2.   The U.S. Department of Health, Education, and Welfare. *(Office of the Federal Registrar)*

are pursued. The following categorical breakdown of organizations in the health system, though arbitrary, attempts to offer a workable framework for discussion. The classification scheme has five basic categories: (1) official agencies, (2) voluntary agencies, (3) professional organizations, (4) philanthropic foundations, and (5) service institutions. Each of these categories will be explained with special attention given to its place in the original activities model.

Official Agencies

The government's interest in health-keeping activities is not new, but the magnitude of its current involvement is unprece-

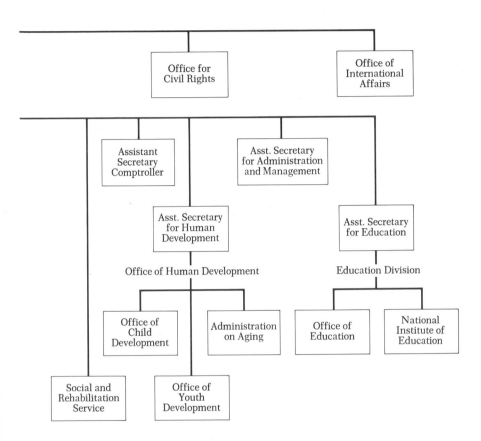

dented. The nature of this work is best viewed through the basic three levels of government: federal, state, and local. The main purpose here is to see the interrelationships among these levels and to understand the basic role of each in the overall health system.

Federal Health Agencies. The word *health* does not appear in the constitution of the United States, and it is only through the broad interpretation of such clauses as "promote the general welfare," found in the preamble, that federal activity in the health matters of private citizens is justified. Yet the actual number of federal agencies involved in various health activities is large, and the growth of this involvement has not been well-planned. As a consequence, for example, much of the drug-control activity is administered through the Department of Justice, while meat inspection is in the domain of the Department of Agriculture. Mine safety is covered by the Bureau of Mines, and certain industrial health standards are maintained by the Department of Labor. In fact, nearly every major department of the federal government is involved in some health-related activity.

This organizational fragmentation has come under heavy attack, and many officials feel that effective functioning is precluded by the lack of overall coordination. In the last several years, various reorganizational plans have been proffered. The ultimate goal has been better coordination among the federal agencies in their health-related activities.

Within this labyrinth of federal organizations, the Department of Health, Education, and Welfare is the most directly involved in health matters. As can be seen from Figure 7.2, it consists of four major branches: Public Health Service, Social and Rehabilitation Services, Social Security Administration, and the Office of Education. Of these, the Public Health Service is the most directly involved in health matters, and the other groups are generally only indirectly active in the nation's health. The Social Security Administration, for example, runs Medicare and its various programs, and the Social and Rehabilitation Service has various programs for the aged and conducts a host of rehabilitation programs. But these instances notwithstanding, it is the U.S. Public Health Service that is most directly involved in the nation's health. Through its Center for Disease Control, it keeps a constant surveillance on disease trends, conducts on-going research in disease causation, and provides the expertise and direction necessary for effective state and local programs. Activities of the Food and Drug Administration provide the framework for the control of harmful substances to which consumers may be exposed and the National Institutes of Health involve a wide variety of research programs in various health matters. These divisions, along with the Health Resources Administration and the Health Services Administration, make the U.S. Public Health Service America's major governmental health organization.

The Public Health Service began as the Marine Hospital Service established in 1798. At that time it served as a hospital service for seamen and was financed by monthly deductions of 20 cents from the seamen's pay. Continuing to grow and develop, the Service became in 1912 the more comprehensive U.S. Public Health Service with responsibility for the health of the nation. Within this century the role of the Public Health Service has expanded as a result of increased government involvement in the health interests of the nation. Each year new legislation is passed which involves the government in greater programs of research, administration, and service related to the health field. Perhaps the major step toward greater federal involvement occurred with the 89th Congress, often referred to as "the health Congress." In 1965 this Congress passed the following laws:[2]

1. Drug Abuse Control Amendments of 1965
2. Federal Cigarette Labeling and Advertising Act
3. Mental Retardation Facilities and Community Mental Health Centers Construction Act Amendments of 1965
4. Community Health Services Extension Amendments of 1965
5. Health Research Facilities Amendments of 1965
6. Water Quality Act of 1965
7. Heart Disease, Cancer and Stroke Amendments of 1965
8. The Clean Air Act Amendments and Solid Waste Disposal Act of 1965
9. Health Professions Educational Assistance Amendments of 1965
10. Medical Library Assistance Act of 1965
11. The Appalachian Regional Development Act of 1965
12. The Older Americans Act
13. The Social Security Amendments of 1965
14. The Vocational Rehabilitation Act Amendments of 1965
15. The Housing and Urban Development Act of 1965

This legislation provided the beginning for what has proven to be an era of increasing government involvement in health matters. In recent times, federal legislation has provided for Comprehensive Health Planning, research on heart disease and cancer, health maintenance organizations, and the protection of the environment through the creation of the Environmental Protection Agency. Still, the greatest illustration of the government's expanding role in the nation's health is presently being debated: national health insurance. Whatever form this legislation ultimately assumes, it will immerse the federal government in the health care field on an unprecedented scale. It would seem, then, that the trend currently and for the future is of an ever-expanding role of the federal government in health matters and, more specifically, increasing work for the Public Health Service.

As its responsibility grew, the Service became a part of the Department of Health, Education, and Welfare. It was incorporated in 1953, and the Public Health Service as well as the whole of HEW have reorganized several times in attempts to provide better for the health needs of the nation.

At the federal level there is much effort in research, program-

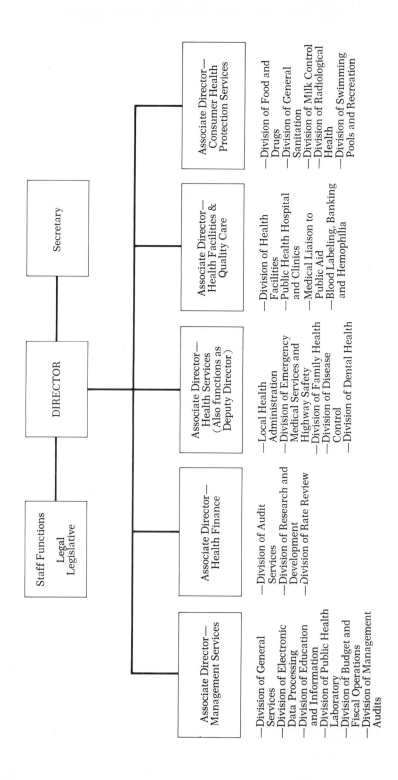

FIGURE 7.3. State Department of Public Health, Illinois. (Courtesy of the Illinois Department of Public Health)

planning, policy-making and the funding of state and local programs. Direct services are provided in part by the Bureau of Health Services to such groups as American Indians, Alaskan natives, prison populations, and merchant seamen. In general, however, the federal government leaves actual program implementation and direct services to the states and, even more, to the local level. In essence there is a division of labor whereby indirect services (research, policy-making, funding) are provided at the federal level, the actual delivery of services is provided by local agencies, and state groups serve as a link between these two levels. This division will be clarified as we explore the roles of official state and local health agencies.

State Health Agencies. Provisions for and the organization of state health activities vary from state to state. Usually the state constitution contains general provisions which the legislature can broadly interpret in order to establish necessary health agencies and programs. This legal framework allows for the flexibility necessary to meet changing health needs.

A major purpose of state health departments is to serve as a link between federal and local agencies. In addition, the state may provide certain direct public services such as immunization clinics, mass screening tests, or well-baby clinics. In most cases, however, the basic purpose of state agencies is to aid local agencies in providing for health needs in the community setting. Figure 7.3 shows a breakdown of one state department of public health. From this diagram it is apparent that the activities of the state health department are diverse and require a considerable amount of manpower and materials. In addition to the state department of health there are other state agencies which perform some health-related activities. Sometimes, however, these create a fragmentation of responsibility and service that is attacked by critics of the health system. Such fragmentation has prompted the recent reorganization of health systems in many states as well as at the federal level.

Despite certain problems, state health departments are indispensable to local community health functions. They provide specialized personnel for advisory purposes, help with needs beyond the capabilities of local health departments, and act as a channel for federal funds and state revenues. The minimum duties of state health departments have been defined by the American Public Health Association as follows:[3]

1. Study of state health problems and planning for their solution.
2. Coordination and technical supervision of local health activities.

3. Financial aid to local health departments.
4. Enactment of sanitary regulations applicable in local health programs.
5. Establishment of minimal standards for local health work.
6. Maintenance of central and branch laboratory services, including diagnostic, sanitary, chemical, biological, and research activities.
7. Collection, tabulation, and analysis of vital statistics.
8. Collection and distribution of information concerning preventable disease.
9. Maintenance of a safe quality of water and the control of waste disposal.
10. Establishment and maintenance of minimal standards of milk sanitation.
11. Provision of services to aid industry in the control of occupational hazards.
12. Establishment of qualifications for health personnel.
13. Formulation of plans in cooperation with other organizations for meeting all health needs.

With the increasing government involvement in health matters, such a listing can be expected to expand. Recently many state health departments have been given duties involving the licensing of some health care facilities for the poor.

Local Health Agencies. It is generally at the local level that direct health-keeping services are provided to the public. With all the research, planning, consultation, and funding at the state and federal levels, the actual results for the consumer are to be found in the programs in the county and community health departments across the nation. It is here that babies are immunized, restaurants inspected, water purified, screening tests provided, the aged visited, alcoholics and mentally ill counseled, and public health education provided. It is in the local health agencies that the elaborate theories and drawing-board programs are subjected to the realities and vagaries of the human condition.

Generally state law dictates that considerable responsibility for local health matters be vested in local agencies whose authority resides in various governmental frameworks such as city, county, or township. Across the nation the actual administration procedures will vary according to locale and particular needs of each area to be served by such health agencies, but usually they are under a local governing body such as the county board of supervisors or a similar municipal body. Often a board of health will be appointed by this

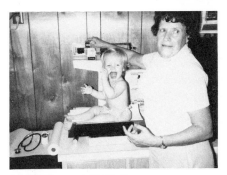

(a) Mother and Child Care

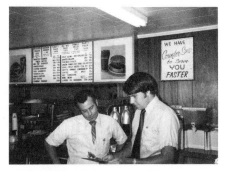

(b) Control of Sanitary Conditions

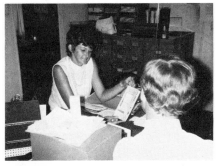

(c) Public Education on Health Matters

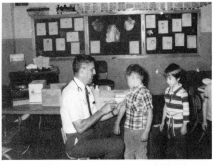

(d) Control of Communicable Disease

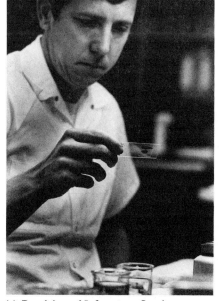

(e) Provision of Laboratory Services

FIGURE 7.4. The kinds of services provided by local health agencies. [*Figures* (a)–(d) *courtesy of the Lawrence County Health Department; figure* (e) *courtesy of Eli Lilly and Company*]

local governing body, and the board will then assume control of the local health agency. It will design the framework, by-laws, and various policies of the local agency and usually be responsible for hiring its director.

As scientific knowledge has expanded, the standard of living increased, and Americans have become more responsive to the needs of others, the demands on local health agencies and their responsibilities have correspondingly increased. Especially within the last twenty-five years it is possible to see significant developments in the areas of psychological and emotional health, public health education, and health services for the young and the aged.

At a minimal level of operation, every local health agency should be active in at least the following areas:
1. Collection of vital statistics.
2. Control of sanitary conditions.
3. Control of communicable disease.
4. Provision of special services to protect the health of mothers and infants.
5. Provision for some laboratory services.
6. Provision for public education on health matters.

These activities are considered basic, and obviously many health agencies go beyond this basic care. Services beyond those listed will be dictated by the special needs of each community setting. Programs for large metropolitan areas or suburban environments will be different both in kind and scope from those in a rural setting. The basic goals, however, will remain the same and only the processes will differ.

Official health agencies thus vary somewhat in their activities at the three levels of government. In relation to the original functional model we can make some distinctions as to the major functions of federal, state, and local agencies.

The federal government appears active in the social policies planning area, for it passes numerous laws, coordinates federal and state activities, sets guidelines for state programs which use federal monies, and generally initiates program and policy ideas to be carried out at the state and local level. Because of its work in such areas as environmental pollution, food inspection, national disease control (through the Center for Disease Control in Atlanta), and consumer protection (through the Federal Trade Commission and the Food and Drug Administration), the federal government would also rank high in the protective activities. Most of this work is achieved indirectly through research, policy-making, and legislation which are then implemented at local and state levels.

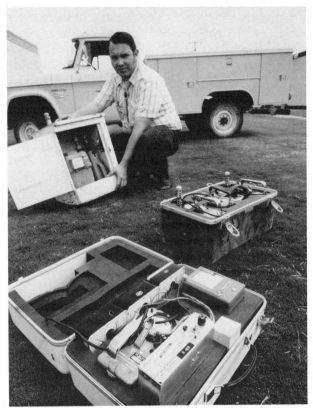

The Environmental Protection Agency is one of the government's most active participant in protective health care. Above is shown mobile monitoring equipment from EPA's Las Vegas National Research Center. The technician holds a portable air sampler; the other instruments measure radiation. *(EPA—DOCUMERICA, Charles O'Rear)*

In the areas of personal care and education and promotion the federal government is not as active. As previously mentioned, it does provide some direct services to special population groups, but generally it gets involved in direct services only when state and local agencies are incapable of alleviating the problem, as, for example, during major disasters.

At the state level there is some activity in each of the functional areas, with perhaps the most emphasis placed on the protective activities and the social policies planning activities. State health departments function in an advisory and coordinating capacity with local agencies, and they provide services where local agencies are incapable or nonexistent. In addition, through state-operated laboratories, legislation, and environmental control measures, they are involved in the protection of state residents. They also do considerable work in the area of rehabilitation, and most states have some institutional services. Thus, personal care activities are a part of their repertoire of activities, although they do not play a major role.

Locally, both the personal care activities and the protective activities have high priority, and education and promotion activities are also given considerable attention. As we have seen, local agencies emphasize such activities as home nursing visits, well-child clinics, screening programs, and immunization procedures. It is on the local level that the real "work" of health maintenance is accomplished.

It must be emphasized that at all levels official agencies participate in each of the activity groupings, but the distinctions lie in the amount and emphasis at each level. The weight assigned in this text can be argued, but the overall distinctions among the three levels are still valid.

Voluntary Health Agencies

Where governmental groups fail to meet the needs of a community or the nation, there often arises a voluntary agency whose pur-

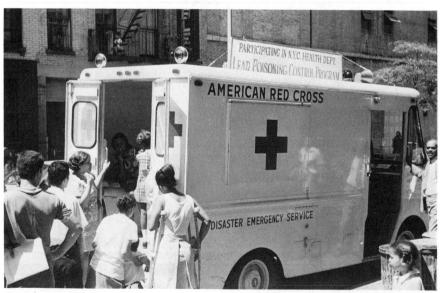

The American National Red Cross is a major health organization that is not a government agency but is also not strictly a private, voluntary organization. It was given a Congressional Charter, and the government directs many of its activities, such as the fulfillment of treaty obligations concerning health care in other countries and emergency health care relief during national and international disasters. Although it is an instrument used by the government to perform various health care duties, it is nonetheless financed by voluntary contributions and staffed primarily by volunteers. *(Courtesy of the American National Red Cross)*

pose is to provide for these needs. Such groups are not tax-supported and are responsible only to their members and public opinion. Most of their funds are raised through public donations, generally in response to yearly organized fund-raising campaigns and constant appeals through the media. Because of their extensive soliciting, most such agencies must be chartered and licensed by state authorities and must meet certain criteria for the chartering process. The actual work and programs of the group are usually governed by a board of directors with members most often chosen from a cross-section of the population.

The voluntary health movement began in this country in 1892 with the Anti-Tuberculosis Society of Philadelphia, which later became the National Tuberculosis Association. When the society was established, tuberculosis was the leading cause of death in the United States, and many people were concerned that not enough was being done to combat the disease. The voluntary agency movement has since mushroomed, and such large agencies as the American Cancer Society, the American Heart Association, and the National Multiple Sclerosis Society have evolved to meet citizen demand that more be done to solve these health problems. In addition to the large national organizations there also exist many smaller agencies often operating at the local level. It has been estimated that over 100,000 voluntary health organizations exist in the United States today.

These voluntary agencies have received both acclaim and condemnation. At times they have proven very effective, as in the case of the Tuberculosis Association in its early efforts at tuberculosis control. In other instances these groups have been of little value. Perhaps the major charge against voluntary agencies is their reluctance to abdicate their role once government agencies develop adequate programs.

Ostensibly, voluntary agencies exist to fill a gap in health programming only until the need is being met by official agencies. Historically, however, voluntary groups have, upon government intervention, simply expanded their programs into other health concerns in an attempt to continue their existence. For example, the National Tuberculosis Association has now become the National Lung Association and concentrates its programs in the broad area of lung diseases, with educational programs regarding cigarette smoking and air pollution. It is often claimed that such situations lead to costly duplication of services and waste of funds, especially in view of increasing government spending on health matters.

It is the public that suffers most of all in this situation, for the citizen is hit financially from two sides. First of all, the private citizen is inundated with contribution requests from voluntary agencies, such as the Christmas Seal drive, the Easter seal campaign, the telethons for multiple sclerosis, and fund-raising campaigns by the Heart Association, the Cancer Society, and the National Foundation. Table 7.1 shows a breakdown of monies collected by these various groups and the obvious magnitude of this collection.

Secondly, a significant amount of the individual citizen's tax dollar is going to government-sponsored health programs which upon close scrutiny seem to duplicate some of the activities of voluntary agencies. Consequently, the public is beginning to ask some serious questions about the raising and expenditure of funds by voluntary agencies and the actual necessity of their existence. For the future it seems that many voluntary organizations will be forced to reevaluate their role and better justify their existence.

Yet there is still a place for voluntary organizations in the American health system, and these groups do have many commendable attributes. One positive aspect of voluntary groups is the involvement of citizens in the solution of a particular problem. The concept of responsibility for the health and well-being of the total community is a positive motivating force, and it gives the individual citizen an opportunity to contribute to the betterment of his fellowman. Such humanitarian commitments can be readily seen in the excellent response to the yearly telethons for multiple sclerosis and other ailments. These activities promote community unity and a feeling of personal worth in relation to group needs.

As noted, voluntary agencies are directed at an unmet need. In recent times these needs have not vanished, they have simply changed. At present, voluntary groups are alerting the public to problems in the areas of conservation and consumer health. Government involvement notwithstanding, it does not seem likely that a time will come when the public does not need to be made aware of certain problems or when these problems do not need to be dealt with before adequate government programs develop. Thus, the role of identifying and alleviating unmet health needs will continue to be a positive role of voluntary agencies.

Another positive aspect of voluntary agencies is their lack of governmental control. Since they are not tax supported, such agencies are not subject to the normal political controls operable in governmental agencies. If their programs are not popular with certain influential groups, less pressure can be brought to bear on voluntary groups than on official agencies whose budget often depends on friendly legislative bodies. As an example, tobacco companies and wealthy tobacco growers can place significant pressure on Congress

TABLE 7.1 The National Information Bureau's rough "campaign" tabulation, February 1974*

Organization	Campaign dates	Fiscal year ends	"Campaign income" only				1973 Support/Revenue		Usual division %
			In fiscal year 1972	In fiscal year 1973	In fiscal year 1969	Compared with 1969 (5 yrs. ago)	Total	% to "research"	N-National L-Local S-State
American Cancer Society	April	Aug.	$ 59,350,000	$ 63,007,000-E	$ 45,559,000	+38%	$ 98,387,000-E	27%-E	40-N; 60-S
American Heart Association	February	June	37,716,000	40,379,000-E	31,591,000	+28%	60,821,000-E	28%-E	25-N; 75-L & S
American Lung Association	Nov. 13-Dec. 31	March	36,090,000	38,005,000	33,437,000	+14%	44,000,000-E	4%-E	9-N; 40-L, 51-S
The Arthritis Foundation	May	Dec.	7,829,000	8,250,000-E	6,484,000	+27%	10,486,000-E	24%-E	35-N; 65-L
Muscular Dystrophy Associations of America	Oct.-Dec.	March	16,607,000-E	17,508,000-E	8,088,000-E	+116%	20,571,000-E	21%-E	75-N; 25-L (Net)
National Association for Mental Health	May	Dec.	10,789,000	12,419,000-E	9,028,000-E	+38%	15,600,000-E	1%-E	7-N; 73-L, 20-S (E)***
National Association for Retarded Citizens	Nov.	Dec.	4,585,000	5,806,000	4,168,000	+39%	7,892,000-E	4%-E	Not Supplied***
Natl. Easter Seal Soc. for Crippled Child. & Adults	March 1-Apr. 14	Aug.	24,525,000	26,000,000-E	19,631,000	+32%	55,000,000-E	1%-E	4-N; 92-L; 4-S (E)
The National Foundation (March of Dimes)	January	May	33,755,000	40,783,000	21,683,000	+88%	43,557,000	5%***	60-N; 40-L (Net)
National Multiple Sclerosis Society	May 12-June 16	Dec.	9,192,000	10,130,000-E	6,120,000	+66%	12,121,000-E	23%-E	40-N; 60-L
Planned Parenthood Federation of America		Dec.	17,300,000	18,400,000-E	13,509,000-E	+36%	42,000,000-E	4%-E	Not Supplied***
United Cerebral Palsy Associations	January	Sept.	16,439,000	18,000,000-E	13,346,000	+35%	27,500,000-E	5%-E	25-N; 70-L, 5-S
Total of 12 National Health Agencies Above			$274,177,000	$298,687,000	$212,644,000	+40%	$437,935,000	14%	
American National Red Cross	Fall & March	June	$118,293,000	$141,850,000	$103,768,000	+37%	$210,889,000	1%	45-N; 55-L (Net)
Local United Way campaigns in U.S.A.	Fall		$858,122,000 for 1973 Expenditures	$918,000,000-E for 1974 Expenditures	$764,327,000 for 1970 Expenditures	+20%			

* The "Campaign Income" figures above are rough totals for the fiscal years noted of "Total support from the public" received directly or indirectly (omitting "Building Funds Campaign," "Special events," "Endowment gifts and bequests," and "Bequests other than endowments") and excluding "Fees and grants from governmental agencies" and "Other revenue." The percentages are very rough comparisons of fiscal 1973 "campaign" results with 5 years ago, and of the ratio of "research" to total 1973 Support/Revenue. There is, of course, duplication in some of the totals above; to illustrate—the American National Red Cross reported recently that about 92% of its contribution income comes through participation in local United Way campaigns. The NIB is a nonprofit organization, founded in 1918, with a twofold purpose: (1) to aid thoughtful contributors to give wisely and (2) to maintain sound standards in its field of philanthropy. (Courtesy of the National Information Bureau Incorporated)

** Exclusive of Salk Institute appropriations of $2,538,000.

*** Distribution varies from chapter to chapter according to percentage based on Effective Buying Income (EBI) as applied to affiliate's area.

E-Estimate

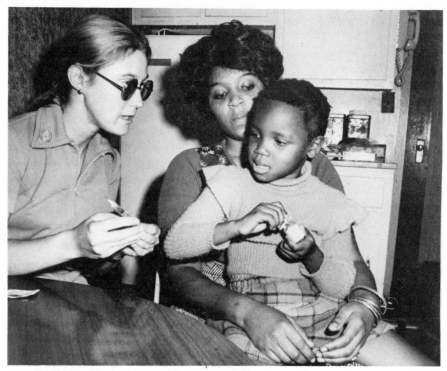

An example of a voluntary, nonprofit organization, the Visiting Nurse Service of New York provides many health care services, including skilled nursing, social work, speech therapy and physical therapy, and an extensive home health aide program. Above, a Visiting Nurse instructs a mother and young diabetic about proper diet and the administration of insulin. *(Courtesy of the Visiting Nurse Service of New York)*

when that body is considering anticigarette legislation. At the same time, the American Cancer Society can pursue an extensive non-smoking campaign with no fear of economic reprisal from tobacco groups. Thus, voluntary agencies can attack a health problem without fear of "stepping on toes" that could result in fund-slashing or a refusal of support. Official agencies, on the other hand, must often modify their approaches to maintain a working diplomacy with those groups which are influential in the outlay of legislative funds. This freedom from political control thus allows voluntary agencies to attack directly major health problems with programs that at the official level might be compromised into ineffectiveness.

In the original diagram of health activities, the major role of voluntary agencies lies in the realm of education and promotion activities. Without exception, the education of the public and community regarding their specific interest areas is a prime function of these groups. In alerting and educating the public about a health problem, voluntary agencies indirectly affect the involvement of official agencies by precipitating public pressure for the government to "do something." Sometimes voluntary agencies also function in the other activities areas, especially the personal care activities. For example, the Easter Seal Society does much work in rehabilitation and provides equipment such as crutches, wheelchairs, and beds for persons in need. The Cancer Society often provides direct services to cancer victims through house visits and rehabilitation counseling. Similarly, some service institutions are founded by voluntary groups.

In summary, the voluntary health movement has been a vital force in the overall health system in America. As health problems change, so will—or should—the agencies themselves. New emphasis, broadened perspectives, and better planning will maintain these agencies as vital forces in the community health field.

Professional Organizations

Most of the health-related professions are associated with an outside organization to which most of the professionals belong. Usually these societies serve to bolster the image, scope, and understanding of the profession both among the professionals themselves and for the general public. Recognizing the importance of competency among their members, these organizations promote continuing education, maintain standards of performance, and work constantly to upgrade the quality of professional education. Through clinics, conferences, conventions and seminars, these groups offer current information to the practicing professional. In addition, they often have committees which set standards of accreditation for schools and colleges. If a college does not meet accreditation, majors from that program will have difficulty obtaining a license to practice.

As with voluntary agencies, there has been a proliferation of professional health groups due, of course, to the expanding field of health and health-related activities. The health professional is inundated with invitations to join this burgeoning list and, inevitably, there is a resultant overlap of functions and fragmentation of efforts to meet professional needs. Such groups as the American Medical Association, American Hospital Association, American Dental Association, American Nurses Association, the American Public Health Association, the Society of Public Health Educators, and the American Association of Health, Physical Education and Recreation give the health professional a smorgasbord of organizations to join. Further, each of these groups has numerous appendage groups which make up the larger whole.

The basic health activities of these professional groups would be found in the education and promotion area. Since their major emphasis is on advancing the profession and ensuring professional quality and competency, these organizations set professional standards, control much of the licensing procedure, and serve as the review mechanism whereby professional incompetence can be corrected. Each professional group recognizes that the quality of the total health system is only as good as the professionals who function in the system.

Because of their influence on the health care system, these professional groups do involve themselves quite a bit in social policies planning activities. Usually they are well represented on boards and policy-making groups and give professional input into decision-making.

Foundations

It has been a windfall for the health field that certain individuals and groups have designated large sums of money to be used for health-related activities. Some of these philanthropic foundations are quite large, with assets in the millions; others are quite small and very limited in funds and purpose. Such large foundations as the Rockefeller Foundation, the Commonwealth Fund, the Milbank Fund, and the Ford Foundation, contribute to a wide variety of causes, among which are health and medicine. Research grants absorb a major portion of this money, but there are also funds provided for individual and public education, and some foundations contribute to the maintenance of institutions to provide care for needy people. At present the entire health field is receiving a great deal of attention from these larger philanthropic groups.

In addition to these larger foundations there are thousands of smaller groups which provide funds for specific kinds of need, many of which relate to the health field. The Rosenstone Fund is a good example of the health interests of these foundations. Its activities include "primarily local giving with emphasis on hospitals and medical research."[4] Similarly, the Elco Charitable Foundation has broad purposes which include "primarily local giving with emphasis on hospitals, community funds and education."[5] These two foundations are representative of thousands of such groups which provide money for research, education, and special uses related to health.

The major health activities of such groups lie in the education and promotion area. In only rare instances do foundations involve themselves in direct services.

Service Institutions

This grouping represents the organizations in the health care system which are most involved in the provision of direct services. Included here are hospitals, nursing homes, and specialized institutions for the care and treatment of people with health problems. Some of these are privately owned, some are government operated, and still others are provided for by volunteer agencies, foundation funds, and private donations.

These institutions basically are involved in the personal care activities. Their structuring is highly variable and they may be governed in a variety of ways, ranging from a board of directors to one chief administrator.

Regardless of ownership or administrative structuring, these service institutions have been receiving special scrutiny in recent times regarding the quality of service they provide. For example, there has been considerable tightening of standards that nursing homes must meet to be licensed and to be eligible to receive medicare patients. Hospitals, both private and publicly owned, are finding consumer groups and government officials more demanding and critical of the quality of the service provided.

Provisions for direct and adequate patient care is the backbone of the health system, and the service institutions provide the setting for this care. Consequently, their role is fundamental, and the current careful evaluation of their effectiveness is only evidence of their importance.

Significant Others

There are still some important groups which are involved in some health activities but which do not fit into any previous groupings. There are many fraternal groups such as Eagles, Elks, Moose, Veterans of Foreign Wars, and Lions Clubs that often intervene to aid needy people in health matters. The Elks sponsor clinics for crippled children; the Lions Clubs provide eye-glasses for needy children; and the Shriners are famous for their hospitals for crippled children. In other instances these groups provide beds, crutches, wheelchairs, and other such equipment for the needy. Most often these services are direct personal care activities and are provided upon demonstration of a real need.

Aside from these groups, there is a large contingent of people and organizations whose involvement in health activities results from the commercial aspects of the health industry. Insurance companies, drug companies, and medical supply groups not only provide some direct services in the health field, but they often involve themselves in education and research programs. The Metropolitan Life Insurance Company, for example, has been one of the biggest producers of health education materials for schools and teachers. Drug companies often produce informational materials and demonstration projects in conjunction with consumer education programs.

SUMMARY

It is impossible to provide a proper categorical niche for every group that might function in some capacity in the health field. The categories presented here do cover by far the largest segment of these groups, but even here there is room for addition and it could be argued that some groups belong in categories other than where they are placed. The main purpose of this chapter, however, has been to provide a working framework, not a complete listing, to aid in the understanding of the organizational complexity of the American health system. Using the functional approach we could examine each category of organization in light of its major activities. Following the categories as presented in this chapter, Table 7.2 identifies where their major contribution lies.

TABLE 7.2   Organizations and their functions in the health system of the United States

Type of organization	Personal care	Protective	Education and promotion	Social policies planning
Official				
Federal	1	4	3	5
State	3	5	3	4
Local	5	3	5	2
Voluntary	3	1	5	1
Professional	2	2	5	3
Foundations	0	0	4	0
		(Research and Grants)		
Service Institutions	5	1	2	1
Significant Others				
Insurance Companies	0	2	4	2
Drug Manufacturers	4	1	2	2
Fraternal Groups	3	1	1	0

Low Input   0 —————— 5   High Input

REFERENCES

1. Mary F. Arnold, "A Social Systems View of Health Action" in *Administering Health Systems: Issues and Perspectives,* ed. Mary F. Arnold, L. Vaughn Blankenship, and John M. Hess (Chicago: Aldine Atherton, Inc., 1971), p. 20.
2. Edward H. Forgotson, "1965: The Turning Point in Health Law—1966 Reflections" *American Journal of Public Health,* LVII (June, 1967), p. 934–35.
3. Lloyd E. Burton and Hugh H. Smith, *Public Health and Community Medicine* (Baltimore: Williams and Wilkins Co., 1970), p. 50.
4. Marianna O. Lewis, ed., *The Foundation Directory* (New York: Russell Sage Foundation, 1967), p. 260.
5. *Ibid.,* p. 227.

SUGGESTED PROJECTS

1. Make a list of health-related agencies in the local area, and then visit selected agencies to inquire about programs, financing, history, and so forth.
2. Take a theoretical health problem and then explore all programs, agencies, and other facilities available to help with that problem. For example, acting as a low-income family with a physically handicapped child, find out what programs, agencies, or other aids are available to help these people. Other examples might include a blind child or persons who need expensive care.
3. Keep a list of health activities recorded in a variety of newspapers and magazines for a one-week period. These activities should then be categorized under the type of organization to which it belongs. For example, if a research grant to study cancer was awarded by the Ford Foundation, this would be listed under the "philanthropic" category.
4. In your free time you might volunteer for a few hours of work with some health-related agency. For example, a local family-planning agency may need volunteers to serve as receptionists. Perhaps a volunteer agency such as the Cancer Society could use someone during their annual campaign. In addition, there are numerous health-related organizations in every community that can always use volunteer help.

8. Community Health Education

Of all the functions of the community health profession, one of the most important has received the least attention. Health education has for decades been in the shadow of large-scale service and environmental health programs, emerging only on occasion in the form of informational programs designed to provide the facts about polio, tuberculosis, and so forth. And even these "tell-it-like-it-is" efforts were sporadic, with little attention given to evaluating their results or to understanding the difference between "health information" and "health education."

Knowing the facts about cardiovascular disease is one thing; behaving in ways that are likely to prevent the diseases from occurring is quite another. And therein lies the difference between health information and health education. The former presents the facts about a health problem; the latter encourages and motivates people to take the information and put it to use—avoiding actions that are harmful and forming habits that are beneficial.

In a medical system that values the prevention of health problems, it is disturbingly paradoxical that while health information continues to grow in volume and intensity of dissemination, health education has been given relatively little opportunity to advance. A great deal of research in the motivation of health behavior has been completed, and more and more health and social institutions are voicing concern about the lack of truly effective health education programs. Yet the implementation of such programs continues to be fragmented and sporadic.

With the exception of a very few states that have enacted progressive legislation for school health education, federal and state support for health education is in lip service only. As shown in

Figure 8.1, of the 90 billion dollars currently being spent for medical and health care, over 92 percent is spent for treatment of existing illnesses. Only about one-half of one percent is allocated for health education. The Department of Health, Education, and Welfare spends about one-fifth of one percent on health education. State health departments on the average allocate less than one-half of one percent to health education efforts.

A major challenge to the community health profession is the extension of viable health education programs to all levels of the community. To be viable, such programs have to be designed to produce desired health behaviors as well as to provide the facts and information necessary for the health consumer to make intelligent decisions. Motivating people to carry out preventive health behaviors and to develop habits that enhance the quality of life are difficult objectives to meet, particularly in the face of the vast number of social and environmental deterrents to the development of sound health behaviors. Nonetheless, the factors that motivate health behavior should be among the criteria used in the development of sound health education programs.

Since its emergence as a viable social institution during the "communicable disease era," public health has been a crisis-oriented profession. Its basic function has been, and continues to be,

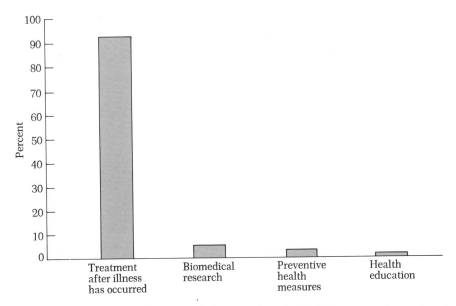

FIGURE 8.1.   Percentage allotments of the approximately $90 billion currently spent each year for medical, hospital, and other health care. (*Adapted from* The Report of the President's Committee on Health Education, *1973*)

the organized response to the health needs and problems of the public, with priorities determined largely by the immediacy and severity of the health problems. Based on decades of experience with health emergencies, the profession has established a substantial repertoire of action programs and a solid reputation for responding to crisis situations with speed and efficiency. Anyone who has witnessed an epidemic of a communicable disease or contamination of a public water supply can testify to the effectiveness of the established procedures for handling these health emergencies.

While the success of these programs can in large measure be attributed to the expertise of the public health practitioners, little could be accomplished without the direct participation and cooperation of the public. A crisis—an immediate, overt threat—is the single most potent factor in motivating direct action by the greatest percentage of the population. Thus, given a logical method of organization and implementation, an emergency health procedure should effectively reach its target population.

As discussed in the previous chapters, however, today's health problems do not constitute emergencies of the direct, overt type. As we shall discuss later, the "diseases" of today are not sufficiently threatening to produce effective health actions by large numbers of the population. The complexities of these problems coupled with our as yet unsuccessful efforts in combating them place an enormous burden on the health and behavioral sciences not only to provide the necessary programs and services but most importantly to stimulate public interest, concern, and participation.

UTILIZATION OF HEALTH SERVICES

Despite the changes in the nature of today's health problems, community health continues to serve its historically defined function: the implementation of programs and services to meet the health needs of the population. In fact, with the accelerating demand for health services of all kinds, there has been a proliferation of health programs on an intensity and scope unparalleled at any other time and place. New health agencies have evolved at the official, civic, and voluntary levels. Traditionally "nonhealth" organizations have taken on health campaigns as their projects for the year—from comprehensive health planning committees to environmental protection agencies to community hot-lines to Girl Scout recycling campaigns.

The success of these programs and services has been sporadic, and in general most programs are at best only moderately successful. Certainly large numbers of people are receiving services, care, and treatment who would otherwise be helpless. In a humanitarian sense, any service that can benefit any number of persons can be termed successful. A more realistic measure of success, however, is in terms of the percentage of a given target population that does *not* participate in, or benefit from, a specific program for whatever reasons. Given this method of evaluation, most mass, voluntary-participation health programs are noted more for their failures than for their successes. Despite massive campaigns, the number of people who smoke, contract venereal disease, abuse medications, do not wear seat belts, do not have cancer examinations, do not receive full-range old-age benefits, are not completely immunized, and so forth, is astronomically high.

Rarely do such programs achieve the objectives set by optimistic community health workers. This is partly a result of unrealistic expectations of the extent to which the public is willing to respond to a "general call"; partly, it is because of the view that some of today's health problems are incurable, unpreventable, and predestined to occur despite measures taken against them; and partly, it is the result of our failure in the community health profession to recognize certain basic concepts of human behavior in relation to disease problems.

It is this last failure that presents the greatest challenge to the community health profession. The availability of community health programs and services is certainly not at issue to any serious extent. It is the public utilization of these programs that represents the crucial problem. We have come to recognize that people do not very often voluntarily participate in a health program simply because it is available or because it appears—at least in the mind of the public health worker—to be the "right and good thing to do." A myriad of forces—cultural, social, community, and personal—stands between the potential consumer of a health service and his utilization of it. To identify these forces, respect their potency, and manipulate them to influence desired health behaviors is a task of great significance to the entire health sciences profession.

COMPULSORY VERSUS VOLUNTARY PARTICIPATION

Much has been said in the preceding chapters about the immensely successful programming campaigns against the major communicable diseases during the 1940s and 1950s. The "formula-success" of these programs is shown by their results. It is certainly legitimate to ask, "If then, why not now?" Why cannot the same procedures and techniques be applied successfully to the health problems of today? The response, of course, is that today's health problems are different—more complex, vague, diffuse, and less well clinically understood. But more importantly, they require a great deal more individual, voluntary action on the part of the public in order to obtain preventive services, care, and treatment. The key elements in the success of communicable disease programs of the past were those that did not rely on isolated, individual decisions but on compulsory behavior or mass, communitywide actions. These elements can be summarized as follows:

1. Legislative activity that required environmental and residential changes such as sanitary waste disposal, restaurant inspections, water treatment, and milk pasteurization.

2. Compulsory activities, often legislative, such as immunizations for school children and tuberculosis testing for specific occupation groups.

3. Community programs carried out with full community support, such as polio immunization clinics and mass tuberculosis screening.

4. Activities that required only a single rather than continuing action, such as immunizations and water fluoridation as opposed to periodic physical examinations and monthly blood tests. However, even single-action activities generally required the presence of other personal motivating factors.

It is important to note that even in those cases where community support was strong but voluntary, individual action was necessary, rarely did the saturation level of the target population reach above 80 percent. Fortunately, communicable diseases can be well contained when only a reasonably large percentage of the animate and inanimate reservoirs of infectious agents has been controlled.

Contemporary health problems do not lend themselves well to compulsory and legislative treatment since these problems are caused more by man's own behavior than by (though often interdependently with) conditions in his environment. Even the most visible environmental problems such as air and water pollution are so closely tied to man's economic and political life that legislation has yet to be successfully enforced in more than isolated instances. As evidenced by the current moral, ethical, and legal controversies regarding drug use, alcoholism, abortion, poverty programs, national health insurance, and birth control, contemporary health issues have shifted in a marked degree from matters of medical diagnosis and treatment to concerns of human rights.

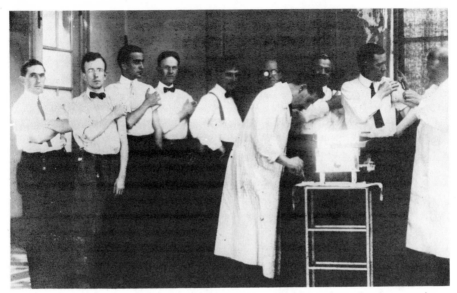

Often influenced more by individual behavior patterns than by pathogenic microorganisms, many of today's health problems do not lend themselves well to the compulsory or quick "shot-in-the-arm" treatment of earlier times. *(National Library of Medicine, Bethesda, Maryland)*

While legislation designed to restrict or compel certain health behaviors will continue to be implemented to counteract severe, overt threats to the nation's health (such as radioactivity), the most powerful determinant of the success of programs aimed at contemporary health problems will be voluntary support, participation, and cooperation at both the community and individual level.

DETERMINANTS OF HEALTH BEHAVIOR

The unpredictable nature of public utilization of health services has been for the past three decades the topic of intensive research in the health and behavioral sciences. Such investigation has been the main reason for the newly emergent professional relationship between these two sciences—the behavioral sciences in their concern with "why people act the way they do" and the health sciences in their endeavor to apply behavioral theories to the design and operation of health programs and services. Just as in the past the health sciences have put into practice medical and scientific principles and discoveries, so do they now apply the concepts and theories of the behavioral sciences—a further "bridging of the gap" which has been the basic operational goal of health education since its professional inception.

A large number of research studies related to the public's health behavior was instigated in the early 1950s, primarily by the Behavioral Science Section of the Public Health Service. These studies were concerned mainly with public participation, or lack of it, in mass voluntary programs such as polio immunizations and tuberculosis screening. Since then, similar studies have been conducted regarding fluoridation, smoking, cancer examinations, stroke rehabilitation, services to the aged, drug clinics, and health insurance. The factors that have emerged from these studies as being the most significant in the determination of health behaviors can be summarized in three general categories: (1) The public's knowledge of specific health problems and programs, (2) community and social forces that influence general support for health programs, and (3) individual perceptions of the nature of health problems and related services.

There is a great deal yet to be learned about human behavior generally and motivation to utilize health services specifically. The above generalizations emerging from recent studies take into account only a portion of the variables that affect program participation. Much has yet to be discovered about the development of health fads, the effects of mass-media programming, effective methods of communicating by motivational techniques such as in commerical advertising, and the public's perception of the role of community health agencies. We know little about public apathy, misinformation, and prejudices in regard to health and illness. Despite the increasing accumulation of behavioral data, the process of decision-making by the "man in the street" that so often produces irrational, impulsive, and dangerous health practices in one situation and effective health behavior in another remains by and large a mystery.

Knowledge and Facts About a Health Problem

It has long been assumed that in matters of health, man is—or should be for his own good—a "rational animal." In other words, given the correct information about a health problem and about measures for combatting it, he will proceed logically and with haste to take advantage of the health services offered to him. This notion has been thoroughly dispelled by several studies which conclude that the "facts" alone are notably ineffectual in motivating changes in health behavior. Few people are unaware of the well-publicized dangers in the abuse of alcohol, tobacco, drugs, and food, and yet the number of people who continue to drink heavily, smoke, abuse medications, and overeat is discouragingly high. Obviously, there are processes and variables that intervene between "knowing and doing," between knowledge and behavior. The community health program that relies solely on broad educational appeals is an example of what has been referred to as the "fallacy of the empty vessel" —community health workers proceeding as if they were pouring their information into a vacuum, void of any intervening factors, rather than into a cultural medium already saturated with existing health attitudes, perceptions, and behaviors.[1] Unfortunately, giving the facts, whether by mass-media bombardment or classroom lecture, is the easiest but most ineffective method of reaching the public. Relating knowledge to action is too complex a process to be achieved in one step, and on occasion is counterproductive when the knowledge is used to rationalize or justify ineffective health behaviors.

This is not to say, however, that knowledge and information have no bearing on health behavior. Clearly, a knowledgeable public is important to the full success of the public health programs, for knowledge is one of the *antecedents* of health behavior for a large percentage of the population. It has been well established that a small percentage of the population responds to health services on

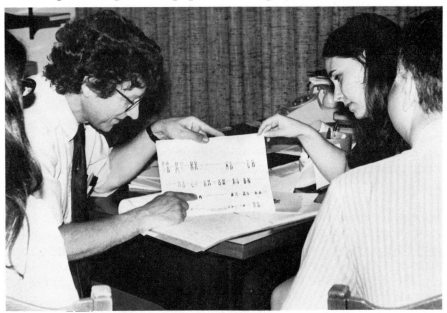

Accurate and understandable information on health matters is essential, though not usually solely responsible, for the effectiveness of health programs. Above, a genetics counselor discusses a chromosome study with a couple concerned about birth defects in their children. *(Courtesy of St. Peter's General Hospital, New Brunswick, New Jersey)*

the basis of rationality alone; an equally small number responds effectively even though completely ignorant of the health problem involved. But the majority of program respondents reveal varying levels of knowledgeability, and their behavior is motivated by a multiplicity of factors. For this reason the function of community health education in attempting to change health behavior is more evident in behavioral research than in works concerned with transmitting facts and information. Clearly, however, the latter do have a place in health programs; it is largely a matter of emphasis.

As Robert D. Russell in his summary of research and writings on the motivational aspects of behavioral changes refers to the fundamental nature of health knowledge: "Knowledge, the main commodity of the educator, is only infrequently a motivator in itself but is an absolute essential when motivation to change behavior is stimulated. The primary responsibility of the profession is still to provide knowledge and learning experiences so that individuals and groups, however they may be motivated, do not lack fundamental facts and understandings as bases for making choices when behavior change seems appropriate."[2]

Community and Social Forces

It has been said, simply and somewhat facetiously, that community health is what the community wants. To accept such a statement is to assume that the community knows what it wants and that what it wants is what it really needs. To deny the statement, however, is to assume that the community as an institution exerts little influence over the programs designed in and for it. Clearly, community forces are decisive factors in the acceptance or rejection, the success or failure, of community-based health programs. Naive indeed is the community health worker whose programming efforts do not pay due regard to the community's formal and informal leadership structure, its sources and distribution of power, and its particular system of organization for the delivery of health care. The political, economic, religious, geographic, and ethnic forces operating within a community define the unique nature and "character" of a specific community, and it is axiomatic that programs of any kind must be designed to fit the profile of the target population.

Because it is not possible in the scope of this discussion to analyze all of the forces at work in a given community at a given time, we will confine our coverage to only two of the major ones: public opinion processes and community subgroups. It is important to emphasize that the public health worker should both respect and understand as fully as possible the unique personality and idiosyncracies of his community.

Public Opinion Processes. Public opinion has always been a crucial factor in the success of community health programs, but never more so than at the present time. With the broad power and scope of mass-media techniques and the "tuned-in" nature of contemporary society, the messages and activities of community health face immense competition from opposing public forces and commerical interest groups. Proper nutrition programs are often effectively countered by private industry's promotion of candy, soft drinks, and convenience foods; the sparing, judicious use of drugs, vitamins, and cosmetics is often successfully opposed by the marketing ploys of the drug and cosmetic industries; the effectiveness of antismoking campaigns is diminished by ingeniously motivating cigarette advertising. Excellent examples of the persuasive power of small interest groups are to be seen in the publicized failures of some proposed fluoridation programs and sex education curricula in schools. These examples underscore the need for community health programs to include in their planning organized attempts to influence, to persuade, to propagandize—in short, to aim directly in as many ways as possible at the opinions, beliefs, and attitudes of the community population. In a very real sense community health must be sold to the health consumer.

Influencing public opinion and collective behavior is a highly complex process about which much is yet to be learned. Our ignorance may be due in large part to the presence and strong, yet unpredictable, influence of such variables as emotions, personal opinions, cultural morals and values, and the many unique economic and political characteristics of a community. Amid the complexities, however, it has been well established that influencing public opinion and motivating collective, community behavior has one common element of particular importance to community health workers—the existence of opinion leaders or "gatekeepers." These are people in the community who have been appointed either formally or informally to serve as go-betweens in the flow of communication from the original source to the general community population. In all groups there exist certain individuals who serve as censors of information and ideas—who learn and pass on information to the rest of the group. Gatekeepers become opinion leaders when they are looked upon by the rest of the group not only as sources of information but as interpreters of issues and purveyors of "expert" opinions and knowledge.

The recognition of this two-step process in communication—from gatekeepers and opinion leaders to community groups—was one of the basic influences in the evolution of the concept of "localizing" the control and administration of many of our federally funded health programs. Comprehensive health programs and poverty programs function under broad federal or state guidelines but require local leadership and control. All employees of these programs are hired by the community, and most of them must be members of the community groups which are being served by the program. In addition, boards of directors and advisory boards are composed of members of various community institutions and professions. Hopefully these people are the gatekeepers and opinion leaders of the community and of the specific groups to whom the services are directed.

The channels through which communications flow in any community or group are specific to that community or group. Many

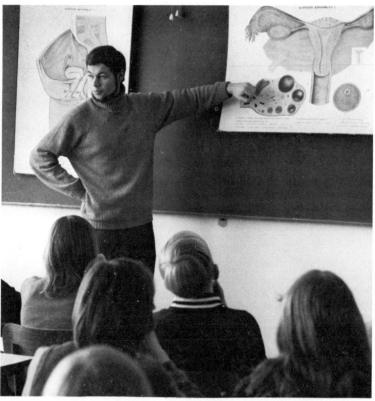

While most people agree that health education should be taught in the schools, there is little agreement over whether sex education ought to be part of that curriculum. *(Courtesy of the World Health Organization)*

studies have revealed a wide diversity, and general lack of consistency, in the processes of communication. Where proposed programs are of a direct medical or clinical nature, such as immunization clinics and epidemic control, health care personnel exert the greatest influence on public opinion. In programs that carry social and moral as well as health connotations, the sources of influence become more diverse and difficult to identify. Individuals with social and moral influence may exist in any stratum of the population, and it has become increasingly apparent that the community health worker must do his "homework" carefully—he must seek to identify and enlist the support of the basic sources of public influence within the community and within specific subgroups of the community. There is greater wisdom in seeking the support of community leaders and strategic individuals than in attempting by mass public health education to obtain the approval by the public as a whole.

Community Subgroups. Among the more important trends in community health in recent years has been the design and implementation of programs for specific population groups within the community: the slum-dweller, the elderly, the handicapped, the overweight, the unmarried, the widowed, and the divorced. While community health has always been concerned with demography (the study of populations subgrouped by age, sex, occupation, marital status, and so forth) in the epidemiological approach to disease control, it has been only recently that we have attempted to develop services based on studies of the social and cultural characteristics of these groups. This trend has developed from our recent rise in "social consciousness," from the public's greater demand for health care, and from the recognition that certain of these population groups are notorious for their lack of utilization of health services.

Along with the recognition of the social nature of today's health problems has come the recognition that an individual's perception and interpretation of health problems and his behaviors toward them are largely a function of the socialization process. While perhaps this does not represent a new revelation to the psychologist and sociologist, it has great significance for the health professional whose basic conern in light of contemporary health problems has been extended from the "habits of health" to the "habits of life."

Socialization refers to the process whereby an individual learns to accomodate his behavior to that displayed and approved by members of the larger social group. The pressures from members of the individual's family or church, his peers in school or work, determine for him what are acceptable and appropriate values, attitudes, and responses. Such pressures of group membership are crucial factors in determining all behavior by the individual, including his health behavior.

In view of these social and cultural influences, it is not difficult to understand the frustrations of the community health wroker who tries to introduce scientific methods amid "folk" attitudes toward illness and medical care procedures among populations who view diseases as the right and just punishment for sinful behavior. Similarly, the difficulties in providing successful programs for lower-income ghetto areas have become evident. The benefits of an increased life span or the prevention of some distant, unknown and

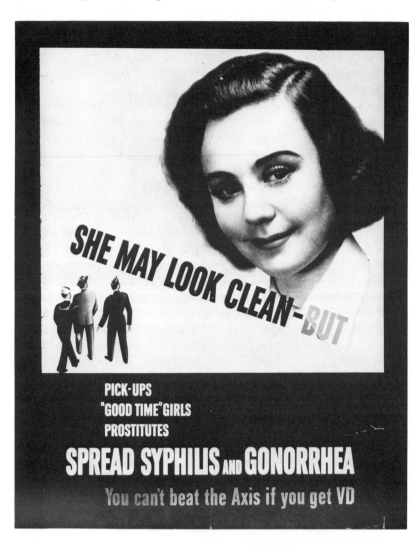

unseen disease become negligible in the face of the more immediate problems of slum life. Studies have indicated that the low-income groups are more likely than other groups to delay seeking medical care and less likely to interpret symptoms as indicative of disease. They are also likely to foster a "folk" approach to illness and medicine rather than a scientific or clinical one. Thus, the cultural gap between the health values and customs of low-income individuals— the group that stands to benefit the most from modern medical care—and those of the traditional health care system continues to widen and thereby contribute to the medical deprivation of the former. In this regard, a question of crucial importance arises: do we as community health professionals attempt to change the slum-dweller to meet the "requirements" of entry into the traditional system, or do we attempt to change the system to fit his social and cultural characteristics?

Health education posters from the 1940s (opposite page) and 1970s (below). Indirectly they illustrate social and cultural attitudes in each period toward a particular health problem. *(Photo opposite reproduced with permission of Technical Information Services, Bureau of State Services, Center for Disease Control, Department of Health, Education, and Welfare; photo below courtesy of The Advertising Council)*

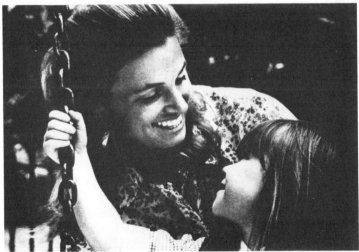

VD is for everybody.

If you need help, see a doctor.

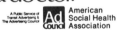

A Public Service of
Transit Advertising &
The Advertising Council

American
Social Health
Association

Another important force molding an individual's actions in accordance with the group's is "social pressure"—the influence which elicits a certain behavior, such as participating in a health program, because one's friends or peers have done so and accept it as "the thing to do." Separate studies by Rosenstock and Johnson and associates concerning participation in polio vaccination campaigns revealed that participation was closely associated with the belief by the individual that others were getting vaccinated and that he himself was expected to join them.

> The respondent perceived friends are his reference group. The actions he believes they took become one basis for deciding what is "the way my kind of people are supposed to act." Thus, persons who believed their friends took the oral vaccine also believed that their friends would approve and praise them for taking the vaccine, too. Similarly, where the persons important to the respondent were believed to have refused the vaccine, the respondent had the psychological experience of group support for his nonacceptance.[3]

In taking this point one step further, Johnson and associates conclude that factual discussions of the dangers of polio and the merits of the vaccine do not seem to be necessary if this type of social pressure exists. "All that appears necessary is for people to have a group of friends and to believe that most or all of these friends will be taking or have taken the vaccine."[4] It would seem that fostering this general impression of group participation would greatly increase the utilization of many types of health services.

A more subtle example of social pressure is seen in the health role expectations of women generally and of mothers specifically. The role of motherhood connotes a health-keeping and protective function with respect to the rest of the family. Thus, women are more likely to participate in health programs and to instigate the participation of other family members because it is appropriate behavior within the context of her family function and not necessarily because of the health values inherent in the action. It is "what every good mother is expected to do" and "what other mothers like me are doing." Similarly, children are expected to care for their elderly parents, teachers for their students, nurses for their patients, and within these roles are potential sources of influence which could stimulate greater utilization of health services.

The influence of group membership and the power of social pressures within the group are promising areas for further study into the motivation of health behavior. Such investigations offer the

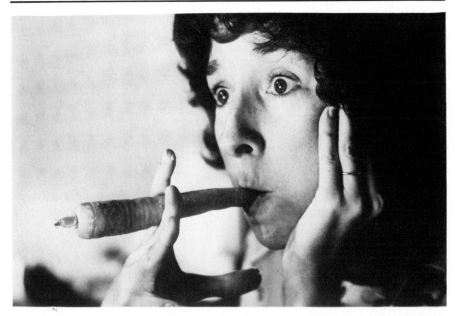

Through its continued efforts in the mass media, the American Cancer Society has effectively been able not only to inform millions of Americans about the dangers of cigarette smoking but also to motivate many to quit. Illustrating the extremes to which cigarette smokers go to fight the habit, the above TV spot, "Ways to Quit," is tagged, "If one of your ways doesn't work, write the American Cancer Society and we'll send you some of ours. We don't care how you quit, as long as you do." *(Courtesy of the American Cancer Society)*

opportunity not only to identify and meet health needs at the "street level" but also to counteract effectively this major weakness in programs whose success depends almost entirely on individual initiative and voluntary participation. The use of group solidarity and social pressures offers the possibility of promoting a kind of group conformity with built-in reinforcement for "good behavior" and social reward for program participation.

Individual Perceptions

The premise that modern health problems require individual responsibilities and actions underscores the importance of understanding the personal element in behavior in relation to both the individual and the group. Any separation of the two is artificial since we are dealing with the individual as a member of a social group or groups. To some extent social influences affect every individual act, and yet an individual must make a personal decision to act even though his motivation to do so comes from the group. However oversimplified, this is the inextricable relationship that exists between the psychological and sociological processes of man. The challenge to the community health practitioner is not to attempt to separate the two, but to determine the relative importance of each in a given setting with a specific health problem existing at a specific time. In some instances personal considerations will be the dominant forces at work; in others, social factors will have greater influence.

A key element in the motivation of an individual's actions is *perception.* We tend to view the world around us subjectively rather than objectively, within the context of our own personal experiences, beliefs, and attitudes. Our perceptions are highly selective and self-reinforcing: we view and interpret surrounding stimuli as we have been accustomed to seeing and interpreting them. In matters of health, our perceptions mold our individual interpretations of the facts and characteristics of a health problem and related health care procedures. We act, or fail to act, according to these perceptions; we observe and listen selectively—out of the myriad of health messages that we receive daily, we will most readily accept those that fit our perceptions on the related health topic. The true facts about any disease may be distorted or blocked out altogether by persons who perceive the disease as a fatal one, an imminent threat, or a social disgrace.

It should be further noted that perceptions are dynamic rather than static states. They are subject to change, and undoubtedly many health programs have been successful in part because they induced such changes. Epilepsy and diabetes are now perceived as diseases rather than inherent "family weaknesses"; mental illnesses are no longer considered incurable; a heart attack victim can return to work rather than live permanently as an invalid.

Although perceptions are highly individualized, it can be hypothesized that a person with a given "set" of perceptions about a health problem and its medical and treatment characteristics will have a *readiness to act;* that is, he will be more likely to do something about a problem if it were to happen to him. Since effective behavior and participation in health programs by the public are the basic goals of the community health profession, the perceptions that constitute a readiness to act are of enormous importance.

The perceptions in this hypothesized set can be labelled as follows: personal threat, severity, salience, high-value priority, and convenience of health services. The person who is most likely to participate in a health program is one who perceives the health problem as being substantially significant in each of these categories.

Personal threat is the degree to which an individual feels susceptible to a given disease, the extent to which he feels it could happen to him, the "closeness" of the disease. As the threat of polio diminished, so, too, did the percentage of people immunized against the disease. Past influenza vaccination programs were often less than completely successful primarily because people felt that neither they nor their families were susceptible to the disease. Young people are not likely to be impressed with prevention programs for heart disease and stroke since these diseases are perceived by them as remote and affecting only the aged.

It is important to note that personal threat should not be confused with fear as a motivating factor. While each has elements of the other, fear is a more highly emotional condition and produces an aura of irrationality that is likely to be a deterrent to effective health behavior. People with a strong fear of cancer, for example, are likely to forego physical examinations, preferring ignorance to the possibility that the disease might be found to exist. Personal threat connotes a reasonably objective and rational view of a disease.

Severity of a health problem refers to the extent to which, should the threat become a reality, the individual perceives the disease would have serious consequences for him. While a disease may be personally threatening to the extent that it is likely to occur, if it is not considered serious in its consequences, the possibility of doing something about it is not as strong. This has been one of the continual problems in controlling the venereal diseases, which are often perceived as "no worse than the common cold." The influenza vaccination programs alluded to earlier suffered from the belief that influenza was at most not much more serious than the usual respiratory illnesses. Serious consequences, of course, may be defined differently by different people—death or disability, pain, loss of income, medical expenses, loss of job, social disgrace, weakness in the eyes of friends, and so forth.

Salience is the benefit, value, or personal reward the individual perceives he will get for participating in a health program. This may take the form of faith that medical procedures will cure the disease, end the pain, extend life, or generally make life more worth living. One of the main problems in treating and preventing many of today's health problems is the lack of complete medical mastery of these problems. "Guaranteed cures" are hard to come by in this day and age, and if the rewards are not perceived as being relatively certain, positive health behavior is less likely to occur. The person whose response to appeals for health program participation is "Why bother?" is obviously unimpressed with the salience of the program.

High-value priority refers to the position of importance that a health problem holds in relation to the other problems that the individual perceives as requiring his attention. If not missing work and losing income is valued more highly than treating a nonacute disease condition that requires hospitalization, then the treatment is not likely to occur. Nor is money going to be spent on health care if there is only enough to cover the bare necessities of living or if social functions or personal habits have greater priority in the family budget or on the family calendar. Procrastination of painful or time-consuming health care procedures is easier if there are other, more convenient or pressing problems to handle first.

Personality characteristics are also potent considerations in the establishment of individual value priorities. Factors in one's personal image, such as strength, beauty, courage, or virility, are often challenged by illness, pain, disability, and the fact that receiving a health service or carrying out a health action might become known to other people. In working with a family-planning clinic in central Ohio, for example, it was discovered that a number of women seeking contraceptive services were prevented from doing so because their husbands considered large families as visible evidence of their masculinity.

Convenience of health services is measured in terms of the amount of effort that the consumer must exert to participate in a health program or service. Health problems lacking in immediate threat and severity can often be approached successfully by making program participation as easy and practical as possible. The success of mass chest X-ray programs was enhanced considerably when mobile units brought the service to the consumer's doorstep. Similar use of mobile units increased the effectiveness of Red Cross blood drives. Many comprehensive health programs provide routinely for transportation to and from the service, baby-sitting, and home visits by health care personnel.

A state of readiness implies a willingness to act, and effective public action is the desired result of any community health program. We have reached the point in community health where we can evaluate the extent to which action is taken by the public, and we have identified many of the factors and processes which influence collective and individual health behavior. The task that yet remains is to put the theory into practice, to develop and refine the techniques of health programming with full recognition of the factors that motivate both group and personal behavior. The need is not only for further research in the motivation of behavior but for more widespread and systematic application of the knowledge we have already accumulated.

SUMMARY

The effective use of behavioral concepts in community health education requires a willingness to go beyond the traditional dissemination of health information. Because of the particular "personality" of a given community, generalized methods of health education will provide only a base level of health information which is at best minimally effective in motivating health behavior. This is not to say that health information is unimportant—on the contrary, it is necessary for the consumer to make intelligent decisions about health matters. By itself, however, such information lacks motivational strength.

The effective application of behavioral concepts in health education has two primary requirements. The first is a thorough understanding of behavioral concepts as they apply to health behavior, both positively and negatively. Much has yet to be learned about the motivation of health behavior, and a great deal of research is currently being conducted on it. The second requirement is a thorough understanding of the community: its people, demographic structure, institutions, and "gatekeepers." Among the first assignments of any community health educator should be a systematic study of the specific nature of his community. Going beyond its history and legal records, the health educator should become involved with, or at least exposed to, as many of its agencies, institutions, and civic and social organizations as possible and as soon as possible. Attempts to conduct programs from offices and through telephone and mass-media contacts are as common as they are ineffective. To effect significant behavior changes requires a commitment to those —and with those—community members and institutions to whom the health programs are directed.

While approaches to health education based on behavioral concepts will have to be adapted to meet specific community characteristics, the following suggestions may provide a point of departure for planning individualized community approaches.

1. Use localized statistics, examples, and health conditions to support proposed health programs. This is necessary for the severity and immedicacy of health problems to be perceived at a local level. Pollution at home now is more threatening than pollution 200 miles away or 50 years in the future; one local fatality in an automobile crash or from a controllable communicable disease usually has more impact than many deaths in another state or country.

2. Stimulate health activity on a group basis to provide social acceptability of health programs. Programs could be designed specifically for family groups, neighborhood blocks, school groups, nursing home residents, occupational and industrial workers, and so forth. Personal contact and direct involvement with the groups to stimulate interest and create social acceptablity are required.

3. Develop and publicize "risk profiles" for various health problems. Identify the demographic and personal characteristics that are related to specific health problems. For example, persons with a high risk of cardiovascular disease are males and females over 50 years old who smoke, are overweight, do not exercise, and have a diet high in saturated fats. Programs available for each profile factor could be included.

4. Use special resource people as leaders or educators in programs designed for specific community groups. Former drug addicts or alcoholics who will speak both objectively and compassionately about their experiences have been effective participants in drug abuse programs for young people. Elementary school teachers could be influential in discussing school health problems with parents' groups. Who can speak with more authority and empathy about poverty than one who is poor? about the problems of senior citizens than a nursing home resident or nurse? about mental health and illness than a "cured" mental patient?

These suggestions are only a few of the many that could be adapted for use in any community. The use of behavioral concepts as guidelines for planning and implementing health programs has much greater potential for behavioral change than the traditional presentations of health information.

REFERENCES

1. Steven Polgar, "Health and Human Behavior: Areas of Interest Common to the Social and Medical Sciences," *Current Anthropology,* 3 (April 1962): 159–205.
2. Robert D. Russell, "Motivational Factors as Related to Health Behavior Change," in *Synthesis of Research in Selected Areas of Health Instruction,* ed. C. H. Veenker (School Health Education Study, National Education Association, Washington, D.C., 1963), p. 108.
3. A. L. Johnson et al., *Epidemiology of Polio Vaccine Acceptance,* Florida State Board of Health, Monograph No. 3, (1962), p. 98.
4. Ibid., p. 91.

SUGGESTED PROJECTS

1. Based on the "perceptions" that motivate health behavior, list the characteristics that would describe the person who is most likely to participate in a program for detecting (screening) high blood pressure.

2. If you were given the responsibility for conducting a cancer detection program in your community or neighborhood, what are the activities or educational programs you might carry out that would relate to the following:
   a. Perceptions of severity and immediacy of cancer
   b. Social group pressure to participate in program
   c. Salience of program participation
   d. Convenience of the program

3. Assume you conduct the program above, how would you evaluate the success of the program? If in your evaluation you wanted to determine the relative strengths of *a* through *d* above, what questions would you ask the program participants? Is it of any value to measure the strength of these items? Why or why not?

4. Prepare a list of periodicals in which research is reported on behavioral concepts related to health behavior. Follow these sources for the next three months and annotate the articles that appear.

9. The Dilemma of Health Care Delivery

It is by now axiomatic that America is suffering from a health care crisis, and anyone who faces a medical emergency, pays a hospital bill, sits in a waiting room, or tries to see a specialist is acutely aware of this fact. Authorities from such varied fields as law, economics, sociology, and medicine are expressing concern over the weaknesses and deficiencies of the health care system; the individual patient is often frustrated and bewildered by what appears to be a nonsystem. The specific problems are many and include fragmentation of services, skyrocketing costs, shortage of medical manpower, lack of quality control, and disparity in availability of services for the poor and the affluent. The literature abounds with reports of needless surgery, misdiagnosis, incorrect therapy, abominable hospital conditions, and medical malpractice suits. The public conscience questions heart transplants and machine survival when children do not get basic immunization and expectant mothers do not have prenatal care. It becomes increasingly difficult to maintain the myth that America is the healthiest nation in the world—especially when it ranks fourteenth in infant mortality, twenty-second in male life expectancy, and eleventh in female life expectancy. Paradoxically, however, America spends more on health care than any other nation in terms both of dollars and of percentage of the Gross National Product. What, then, is the problem with health care in America?

It is the purpose of this chapter to view some of the answers to this question. Initially, the focus will be on the factors which combined to precipitate the current crisis. Attention will then be directed to those specific issues which appear the most formidable at the present. Obviously, within a system all elements are interrelated and it is not possible to isolate one aspect of the health care system from the other elements in that system. This fact will become readily apparent in the following pages.

PRECIPITATORS OF THE CRISIS

Societal problems that reach the crisis stage are not the result of some spontaneous combustion, but rather have evolved over a period of time. Accordingly, the current problems of the health care system have developed through time from a variety of concurrent and interrelated factors.

Paramount among such factors have been the dramatic ad-

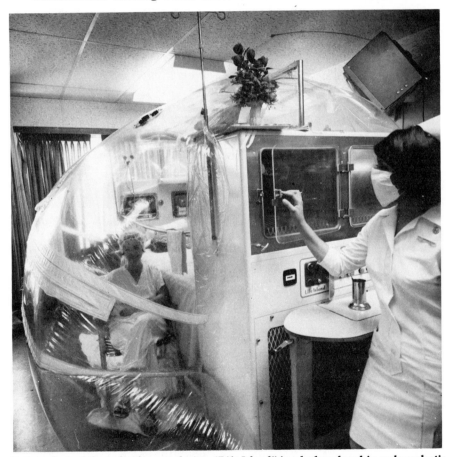

One product of the technology explosion, "Life Island" is a bed enclosed in a clear plastic bubble designed to provide patients under high dosage of anti-tumor medications with a sterile environment. *(Courtesy of the World Health Organization)*

vances in medical technology. Even the casual observer of the mass media is aware of heart transplants, kidney machines, plastic surgery, new vaccines, and the latest in cancer therapy. Diagnostic and therapeutic techniques develop at a mind-boggling rate with each new discovery, demanding greater outlays of money and manpower. Electronic devices, nonexistent fifteen years ago, are now standard equipment in many hospitals. It has been observed that "in one recent five-year period the number of laboratory procedures commonly carried out in hospitals tripled, creating a demand for all kinds of arcane instrumentation."[1] Surgery and its techniques have advanced to a degree that organ transplants, open-heart surgery, and donor banks are everyday terminology even to the layman.

The artifacts of modern medicine are impressive indeed, even perhaps a little frightening. Yet a closer observation will reveal an even more astonishing element about this technology—the speed of its development. Not more than fifteen years ago there was little thought of cobalt machines, pacemakers for the heart, instruments for the removal of cataracts, artificial heart valves, and such attendant problems as the precise determination of death and the morality of sustaining terminal patients and defective newborns. The prognosis for diabetics was bleak before the discovery of insulin in 1923, and only since the 1940s has penicillin been available as the principal drug for a host of bacterial agents. Through the recent innovation of amniocentesis it is now possible to determine the sex of the child in utero, as well as his chances for physical or mental defects; following birth a battery of tests is available, including a new test for P.K.U.—a metabolic disease resulting in mental retardation.

The above list is only a sample. Each day the efficiency and scope of medical know-how increases perceptively, and each new discovery, when added to the existing technological pool, is a potential precursor of a multitude of dramatic breakthroughs in medical science. Consider, for example, what the understanding of the body's immune system has meant for the development of more effective vaccines, the ability to combat the rejection syndrome in organ transplants, current efforts to find a viral cause of some cancers, and the control of severe allergic responses (anaphylaxis) due to the increasing number of chemicals in the environment. In like manner the discovery and identification of various hormones, when added to previous knowledge, has provided both birth control pills and fertility drugs as well as the ability to control numerous conditions resulting from hormone deficiencies.

Each of these developments, while adding to the field of knowledge, is built on the accumulated knowledge up to that point. This accumulation process occurs in such a way that the knowledge doubles and quadruples within increasingly shorter intervals, and so a discovery, requiring twenty years for fruition at an earlier time, now happens in five years. Consequently, the most inspiring achievements in medical knowledge and technology have occurred in this century, and changes and new advances continue to occur at an accelerated pace. This explosion of knowledge and technology has been put in perspective by one observer of the medical scene:

> Somewhere between 1910–1912 in this country, a random patient, with a random disease, consulting a doctor chosen at random, had, for the first time in the history of mankind, a better than fifty-fifty chance of profiting from the encounter.[2]

In fact, the view that medical science has the potential to solve all of man's ailments is dated within this century, probably within the last three decades.

Out of this view emerges another factor which has done much to precipitate the current health care crisis: a rising expectation level on the part of the individual. The significant improvements in the quality of medical techniques have been accompanied by increased expectations in the quality of health itself. Ailments that were tolerated at earlier times now become a matter of medical concern demanding physician intervention. Consequently, the health care system is being utilized for the treatment of many ills which are borderline and could be handled by paramedics rather than physicians. In addition, modern medical improvements have significantly lengthened the life span of many, creating an increased demand in health care for the aged. More is now being demanded from the health institutions than they are capable of providing, and thus they fail to meet the expectations which their very successes have created. Americans have become accustomed to the "good life" whose amenities include the somewhat utopian state of perfect health, and this attitude combined with the increasing faith in medical "fix-it" techniques presages a continuing burden on the present health care system.

Closely allied with rising expectations is the current belief that good health is an inherent right of man, not the exclusive domain of a privileged few. Given American democratic principles, the demand that access to health services be equitable for all is not an unapproachable ideal. But given the high level of health care possible, it may be economically and physically unfeasible to provide the "best" health care for all people. Although human idealism would have the migrant worker be given the same care as the bank president, it is impossible for every physician, clinic, and hospital to be the "best." Perhaps the concept of "best" should be replaced by "adequate," for realistically the current demand for equal health care may prove feasible only in the sense of adequate care for all, and medical miracles may remain possible for only a chosen few. Yet meeting even an adequate level will prove difficult for the current health care system, and it is this goal which will be a driving force in future programs of health care.

At this point it is important to note that the actual organization of the health care system itself has fostered a major part of the health care crisis. Composed of a multitude of agencies, practitioners, and facilities, the system is fragmented into diverse pluralism which alienates patients and precludes adequate care. For every disease there is a specialist; for every need a separate clinic. From gynecologist to pediatrician may be across the hall, across town, or across county. Seeking health care is a selection process from a smorgasbord of acute hospitals, family-planning clinics, rehabilitation centers, mental health centers, drug rescue groups, private physicians, and a host of voluntary and professional groups. Under these circumstances comprehensive and continuous care is not possible, and the patient feels frustrated at being at the mercy of the medical complex and often loses a sense of identity so important to medicine as an art.

The culprit here is poor organization. Efficiency experts are appalled at the lack of productivity from the medical care arena, and to them its disorganization is frightening. For the individual patient as well as the total health care system, a reorganization is not only necessary now but would appear to be the sine qua non of any effective health care in the future.

Thus, the health care crisis is the product of many forces interacting in concert and impinging on an entity which has developed haphazardly with little or no direction—namely, the system of health care delivery. Many of the inadequacies are evident; some as yet unnoticed are beginning to emerge. It is these specific problems and issues which will be the concern of the following pages.

INEQUITIES IN HEALTH CARE

For the poor, whether black or white, young or old, health care is at best a degrading, dehumanizing experience with long waiting periods, impersonal care, charity overtones, and poor accessibility; at worst it is a nonexistent entity precluded by cost and availability. For many Americans, basic preventive measures such as immunizations and medical check-ups are as alien to their personal experi-

ences as space walks to the average citizen. While medical specialists and skilled technicians work feverishly to maintain a comatose
octogenarian, there is a malnourished Appalachian child, a migrant
family with typhoid, or a poor elderly black with emphysema who
may wait for hours to see an overworked and ill-equipped physician
in a remote area devoid of even basic nursing aid. For those who can
afford them, advances in medical care are a real boon; for those who
cannot afford even minimal medical attention, there still remains
a great gap between the actuality and potentialities of health care.

The relationship between poverty and ill-health is well established, and admittedly much of the problem is a reflection of the
total aura of poverty, including poor nutrition, lack of education,
inadequate housing, unsanitary living conditions, and overall life
style. This is only a partial explanation, however, for there also
exists an obvious shortcoming in health care available to the poor.
While utilizing medical facilities much less, the poor show greater
severity of illness and longer hospital confinements than the more

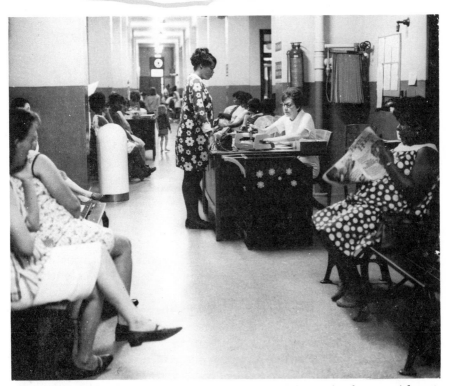

Public health clinics are the second major source of health care for the poor. Adequate
medical treatment is usually provided, but often only after long waits in uncomfortable
surroundings. *(Courtesy of the World Health Organization)*

fortunate of society.[3] The longer hospitalizations can be partially explained by the lack of early medical intervention which would preclude the need for hospitalization in the case of many ailments. Explanations for this lack of preventive treatment include cost, accessibility, and quality in the health care of the poor.

For the poor, which includes many minority groups and large segments of the elderly population, the private practitioner still serves as the major link with the health care system. The relationship here is not, however, consistent with the traditional concept of the personal physician who provides continuous and comprehensive care for his patients over long periods of time with much personal knowledge of family and social backgrounds. On the contrary, such a close, long-term relationship is a rarity between the poor patient and his doctor, and low-income families, as well as older medicare and old-age assistance patients, seldom have one doctor over long time-periods to whom they can turn with all their health problems. In addition, the situation is aggravated by the fact that the social backgrounds, experiences, and values of the doctor and of his poor patients differ so greatly that the physician is often very reluctant to initiate a close relationship with them.[4] Yet this does not lessen the need for practicing human medicine as an art with concern for the total patient rather than just for the biological part that is diseased. Whether poor or rich, filthy or clean, beautiful or unsightly, humans are psychological beings who require understanding beyond the sterile approach of antibiotics, needles, and X-rays.

Yet given the shortcomings of the relationship between the poor and private practitioners, this relationship has advantages over the public clinic where the impersonal approach is most evident. These clinics serve as the second major source of health care for the poor, and the poor—welfare recipients, minority groups, ghetto-dwellers, the unemployed, and the elderly poor—represent the major patient population of these clinics. Consisting of outpatient departments, emergency room and public health clinics, these facilities usually provide adequate technical treatment, but they are consistently condemned for an organizational pattern which is convenient for the providers but which, through its fragmentation and neglect of social considerations in the treatment of an illness, is disastrous for the patient. Seldom is the clinic designed to provide even minimal comforts for the patients, and the low status of such clinics in the eyes of health professionals prompts an aloof indifference to the humanness of each patient. Consequently, scientific treatment for the poor may exist, but the setting for its administration and actual delivery does not resemble the type of medical art available to the more affluent.

At this point, it may still be debated whether or not "health is purchasable," but it seems obvious that health care is at least more easily obtained by those who have the finances. For substantiation of this point it is helpful to view the institutional setting—the hospital—for a comparison of treatment between the poor and those of better means, essentially a comparison between private rooms and ward accommodations since such distinction is determined on an economic basis.

Studies indicate that many hospital wards are outdated, dismal, and inadequate to meet the standards of good health care. Again, the major shortcoming is not necessarily inadequate technical care but a detached, impersonal approach to the patient and his human needs. Alienation best describes the lower-income patient's feeling about his hospital treatment, which usually exhibits little concern for his overall needs. This fact was given credence in the study by Duff and Hollingshead of one major hospital ward.

> For the most part, the physicians were not able to identify with these patients. To be well, young, and vigorous was to be in a very different position from that of an older, sick, or dying patient. The future of ward patients was usually dismal; that of their sponsors offered an extreme contrast. The young physicians looked with anticipation toward a career in medicine. They hoped for the time when they would not have to do such work and associate with "crocks" and "crud." Meanwhile, they learned in the ward accommodations but indicated their awareness of the patients' situation in various ways such as naming these wards "the zoo."
>
> Although the ward patients were silent about their treatment, they were often seething with anger. When they told us their stories, we had to cope with the resentment of persons who were often depressed and suspicious. They asked us why we didn't "do something" about their situation instead of "wasting time asking questions and doing studies." We could only answer that we hoped this was a beginning. (It was not a satisfactory answer to the patients, and the researchers often felt acute embarrassment.)[5]

These inequities in health care treatment can be further seen in the plight of the elderly poor. At a time when increasing numbers are living well after retirement, the health care system seems increasingly unable to provide for the continuous, long-term care necessitated by the ailments characteristic of old age. Especially dismal is the outlook for those whose savings or insurance benefits are inadequate to meet the cost of long-term care. Medicare, Medicaid, and Old-Age Assistance have proved only partial answers and in many ways have increased the problem by encouraging profit-motive nursing homes and yet lacking effective control over the quality of care provided by them. Further, government payment for nursing-home care is relatively low and has tended to induce poor treatment. With reports of inadequate conditions in many nursing homes, however, government officials have balked at increasing payments. This witholding of funds in turn tends to perpetuate inadequate care since profit-oriented firms must either cover costs or keep their services at a minimum. Consequently, the situation

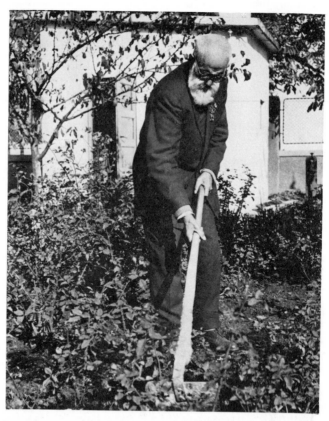

Recent medical advances, which have lengthened the life span of many, have also created an increased demand in health care for the aged that is difficult to keep pace with. This man, 116 years old when the photograph was taken, is shown working in the garden at the Geriatrics Institute in Bucharest. *(Courtesy of the World Health Organization)*

exists in which nursing-home owners refuse to upgrade their care until more money is made available by the government, and the government refuses to pay more until the care is better. In dealing with this problem one nursing-home administrator has offered his solution to costs: "use fewer nurses and replace them with tranquilizers."[6]

Positive efforts notwithstanding, there simply has been little long-range planning to meet the problems of old age. Indeed, many experts agree that a substantial portion of the nursing-home population (perhaps 15 percent) could be cared for at home through a home health program utilizing visiting nurses. Yet there has been little funding for such a program, and many of the aged, especially the poor, continue to be subjected to needless institutionalization in demoralizing "prefuneral homes."

There appears to be a dual system of health care: one for the haves and one for the have-nots. The dichotomy between these groups is far from distinct, however, and in reality it involves a continuous line from the totally indigent to the very rich, the mass of society falling along the continuum. Where does one have to fall along this line to be unable to afford health care? The answer is uncertain, but as costs increase, the cut-off point moves more and more in the affluence direction. Herein lies a haunting spectre of the health care system, for who can say who will be the have-nots—in a medical care sense—in the future. Humanitarianism aside, it behooves the affluent of society to correct the current inequities of health care from the standpoint that monetary considerations may, in the future, preclude adequate health care even for those who are well-to-do. Realization of this point may in fact prove a better motivator of positive action than the current appeals to the humanitarian principle of good health care as a basic right of the individual, for it appeals directly to the basic idea of self-preservation.

THE COST EXPLOSION

Thus we come to a second major element in the health care crisis: mushrooming costs. Precipitated by a variety of forces, this aspect of the current dilemma is perhaps the most discussed since it involves all segments of the population and thus has greater mass media recognition. The inflationary spiral includes physician fees, hospital costs, and drug prices which together make health expenditures one of the major contributors to the overall cost-of-living increases. The statistics are staggering. As can be seen from Table 9.1,

TABLE 9.1   Average annual percent increase in cost of living and medical care*

Year	Consumer price index, all items	Medical care
1946–60	3.0	4.2
1960–67	1.6	3.2
1967–71	4.8	6.6
1966–67	3.0	6.5
1967–68	3.3	6.4
1968–69	4.8	6.5
1969–70	5.9	6.4
1970–71	5.2	6.9

* From the U.S. Department of Health, Education, and Welfare.

the cost of health care has risen much faster than the cost of living, thus negating the view that health costs are a simple reflection of price increases in the general economy.

Consistent with this observation one finds a concomitant increase in the percentage of the Gross National Product spent on health care. Figure 9.1 shows the dramatic change from 4.6 percent in 1950 to 7.6 percent in 1972, which amounts to a raw dollar difference of nearly 72 billion dollars. The 83.4 billion dollars spent in

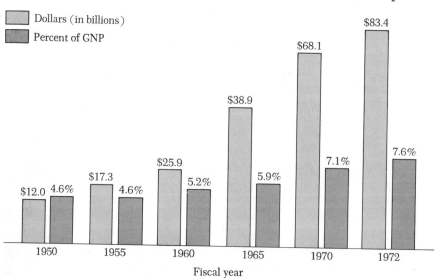

FIGURE 9.1.   Today's medical care dollar totals $83.4 billion: 7.6% of the Gross National Product. (*Office of Research and Statistics, U.S. Department of Health, Education, and Welfare*)

1972 represented an outlay of 340 dollars for every person in America. Yet if this seems awesome, consider the projection for the year 1980 which indicates medical care expenditures will total 189 billion dollars, with each American having a health bill of 814 dollars.[7] Further consider one estimate that by 1980 the cost of staying in a major urban teaching hospital will be as much as 1,000 dollars per day, and in a community hospital it will be about 500 dollars per day.[8]

At this point it is clear that the cost-rise cycle will necessarily continue, but the speed and magnitude of this rise is not unalterable and herein lies the possibility for ameliorative action. The basis for such action comes from an analysis and understanding of the economics of the health care system with its unusual characteristics that often defy adherence to basic economic laws.

From the economists' standpoint, the health care industry enjoys a unique place in the concept of a free-market economy. Based on the idea that competition works to control prices, such a system allows consumer choice to force producers (providers) to sell their product at the lowest cost. In health care, unlike other goods and services, the consumer is in a poor bargaining position based on his own needs (often immediate), lack of competition (based on an obvious monopoly), and little consumer knowledge (did I get a good deal?). In essence, the health care system is a seller's market where "all the traffic will bear" is all too often a reality. This situation is exacerbated by the traditional economic law of supply and demand, for the demand for physician services is currently exceeding the supply, thus inducing cost increases for a limited commodity.

The shortage of physicians is a major element in the total health care problem, but it must be kept in perspective or else solutions to the overall health care crisis become difficult. For example, if all efforts to relieve the shortage are directed toward simply preparing more physicians, the end result at best would be a maintenance of the status quo. The fallacy of this approach is obvious if one realizes that if every medical school immediately doubled the size of its freshman class, in eight years there would be 16,000 new doctors as opposed to the current 8,000 per year. But as much as 25 percent of these young doctors choose not to get involved in direct patient care, and thus by 1990 there would be an additional 78,000 practicing physicians.[9] At the present level of physician productivity this increase would still prove inadequate. Of course, the original thesis is untenable since medical schools simply are not equipped to handle such an influx of students, the basic limitations being teaching manpower and physical facilities. Medical schools should be encouraged to increase their manpower output, but "a realistic goal of an immediate 10 percent increase in medical school enrollment would add only 7,800 extra physicians to the national pool by 1990."[10]

A more feasible approach to the physician shortage and concomitant cost increase is a greater level of productivity from the present practitioners. Increasing physician productivity is not just a matter of longer hours, however, since most physicians already work well beyond an average work week. Rather, an increase in productivity lies with the effective utilization of allied health personnel to whom selected activities can be delegated in order to release physician time for more specialized tasks. Utilization of such individuals who require less expensive training would cut down on the waste of the more expensive physician time while allowing for the treatment of more patients. The Medex Program operating in

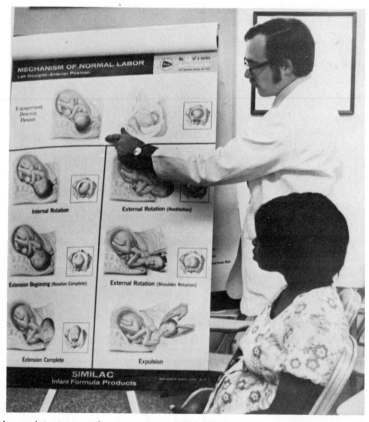

Physician assistants can take over many of the tasks formerly performed by the physician, thus freeing the physician to employ his more specialized talents. Above, a physician assistant explains the growth of the fetus to an expectant mother. *(Courtesy of the Bureau of Health Resources Development, National Institutes of Health)*

the state of Washington is a good example. A joint effort by the University of Washington and the State Medical Society, the program originally enrolled 15 former military corpsmen in a three-month training course and then placed them in one-year apprenticeships with rural physicians. Under supervision the trainees treat children's respiratory infections and lacerations and aid in surgery where normally two doctors are needed. According to one cooperating physician, the hiring of one trained corpsman will allow him to see twenty additional patients per day.[11] Similar programs are being pursued in other parts of the nation and presage a tenable alternative to increasing the number of physicians in order to increase productivity.

Beyond the manpower issue lies another possibility for productivity increases: mechanical devices. Computers have proven valuable in the quick interpretation of medical histories, the reading of electrocardiograms, and diagnosis of illness based on the symptoms and syndromes presented to it.

Yet in each of these possibilities, the physician remains the central determinant. Unless the medical profession accepts these alternatives, they have little chance of fruition. A computer not used, a trained army corpsman unhired, or a pediatric nurse given few duties beyond bottle-sterilizing can do little to solve the problem. Essential to greater medical system productivity is the acceptance by the medical profession that there are viable alternatives to the increase of practitioners as a solution to the health care crisis. The challenge to the physician is to seek and utilize these alternatives.

The physician is further implicated in another money-wasting aspect of the health care crisis: the time-honored but now archaic fee-for-service system. Most economists are vigorous in their criticism of this system and feel it is the major flaw in medical care today. This criticism is not new, but it is increasingly vehement. They point out that under such a system the doctor gains economically from the number of patients he sees and the amount of expensive procedures he employs. The patient's interest is therefore in conflict with the doctor's economic needs to see more patients and treat more problems. Consumer groups as well as many medical professionals are aware of this situation and a change seems imminent.

Still, if one looks closely at the health care dollar, physician costs consume significantly less than do hospital costs. Hospital costs have risen much faster in recent times than have physician fees. From 1967 through 1971 the average annual increase in hospital daily services charges was 13.5 percent; the same average for physicians' fees was 6.7 percent. Behind this trend are such factors as technical equipment, unnecessary hospitalization, increasing consumer demands, third-party payments, poor management, and general system weaknesses which result in inefficient and ineffective usage of hospital beds. Although the solutions proferred are manifold, they all revolve around two basic possibilities: lower the cost of the hospital or decrease the use of its facilities. The former is laudable but highly unlikely given the cost-of-living increases and continual development of expensive technology. The latter is more feasible and involves a continuance of the present overall assessment and restructuring of the total health care system.

Before leaving the cost element, two further factors must be considered: the impact of health insurance and the medical-indus-

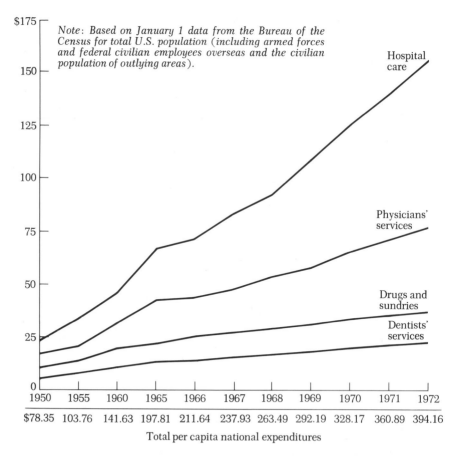

FIGURE 9.2.   **Per capita expenditures for health care, selected items, fiscal years 1950–1972.** (*From Committee for Economic Development,* Building a National Health Care System. *New York: Committee for Economic Development, April 1973*)

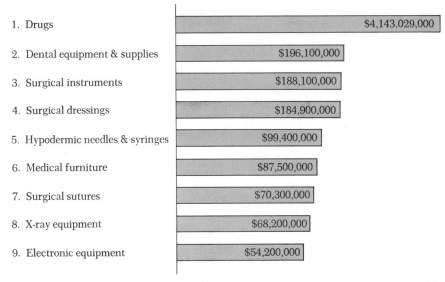

1. Drugs — $4,143,029,000
2. Dental equipment & supplies — $196,100,000
3. Surgical instruments — $188,100,000
4. Surgical dressings — $184,900,000
5. Hypodermic needles & syringes — $99,400,000
6. Medical furniture — $87,500,000
7. Surgical sutures — $70,300,000
8. X-ray equipment — $68,200,000
9. Electronic equipment — $54,200,000

FIGURE 9.3. **Value of manufacturers' shipments of medical supplies.** (*From Harold B. Myers, "The Medical-Industrial Complex," Fortune (January 1970): 91. Bob Weiss Associates for Fortune Magazine*)

trial complex. A great deal of data has been collected which indicates that third-party payments* have encouraged both doctors and patients to overuse health care. With the advent of Medicare there was a documented increase in the cost of care for the elderly at all levels of the health care system. In 1966, just one year prior to the beginning of Medicare, each individual directly paid 51 percent of his bill, which averaged out to 94 dollars. By 1972 the individual was paying 119 dollars, but this represented only 35 percent of his bill. Some evidence indicates that if the patient is covered by insurance, even the most reputable physician may prescribe diagnostic tests and medical treatment to a greater extent than if the patient had to pay his own bill. Health insurance may also induce the doctor to allow the insured patient a few extra days of hospital care to ensure a total recovery. The situation is further aggravated by the fact that insurance companies have tended to pay only for inpatient care and thus have encouraged the hospitalization of patients who could be adequately cared for on an ambulatory outpatient basis. Thus it may be justified to say that what most Americans have is sickness insurance and that comprehensive health care at a reasonable cost is not yet a reality. And yet if there is an increase in coverage, premiums will necessarily go up unless government, consumers, private insur-

---

* Payments from sources such as Blue Cross, Medicare, and so forth.

ance companies, and the medical profession join in solving this aspect of the cost-rise dilemma.

Finally, some attention must be given to the medical-industrial complex as a factor in health care costs. This complex involves the manufacture, sale, and distribution of the various supplies needed by the health care industry. Figure 9.3 gives a sample breakdown of the kinds of supplies needed. From this figure it is not hard to understand why hospital supplies and medical electronics were the glamour stocks of 1969 and 1970.[12] Consider not only the increases in over-the-counter and prescription drugs but also the amount of disposable needles, bandages, scalpels, and gloves as well as the new equipment and needed furniture—it is an entrepreneur's utopia.

Amassing great profits from supplying the growing health care market, companies in this field have a big stake in the health care system. They will no doubt be a powerful voice in future attempts to alleviate the current cost problem.

QUALITY OF CARE

Closely aligned with the growing discontent over its inequities and high cost is the rising dissatisfaction with the quality of health care. Both health care professionals and consumer groups are voicing concern over the type of health care offered by some segments of the health care industry. Increasingly aware as well as expecting more in health matters, today's health consumer is demanding a greater accountability from the health professions. In some instances consumers are vehement in their condemnation of the care they are receiving. The problem arises from two broad areas of concern: (1) the professional-technical aspects of care, and (2) the psycho-social context of providing this care. The former involves physician competence, institution quality, and the technical aspects of the care provided; the latter involves those elements which make health care accessible, desirable, and responsive to the individuals it serves.

The responsibility for the quality of health care has traditionally been left in the hands of the health professions. According this group much respect and considerable power, society has tacitly expected the profession to ensure the good conduct and competence of its individual members and institutions. Current efforts are directed toward the development of exact standards and policies to police the competence and quality of health care professions.

There are, nonetheless, recorded instances of needless surgery, misdiagnosis, improper medication, and professional ineptitude. In a study of perinatal mortality it was found that 44 percent of deaths in mature infants and 29 percent of deaths in premature infants were associated with preventable factors. Errors of medical judgment were found operable in 80 percent of these deaths.[13] Table 9.2 shows the results of a study on the justification of surgery and reflects the influence of the method of payment and type of hospital on the incidence of possibly unnecessary surgery. Interestingly, even in the best hospitals with seemingly the highest standards, approximately one-third of the primary appendectomies were not clearly justified. And these statistics do not even account for the errors of omission, which doubtless occur, where needed surgery is not performed and the patient suffers accordingly.

From the numerous studies on the quality of services there emerge basic commonalities. In general, services of poor quality are found more frequently in certain types of institutional settings and as given by certain categories of physicians. It should not be construed that poor-quality care is equally distributed throughout the health care field. On the contrary, the best care has been found in those hospitals affiliated with medical schools, and the poorest care has been uncovered in unaffiliated proprietary (for profit) hospitals. The worst physician performance was found among physicians who were not specialists and who practiced only in proprietary hospitals. Seventy-one percent of these physicians' cases were rated as having less than optimal care.[14] Such data indicate the possibility of identifying high-risk settings for poor-quality care, and further imply that the study of the quality of services is an important area of investigation for the improvement in general of health care delivery.

Many factors are involved in medical care quality. The recruitment and training of good personnel is a primary consideration.

TABLE 9.2   Percent of appendectomies that are unnecessary or doubtful in university and community hospitals*

Pay status of patients	University hospitals	Community hospitals
Welfare (N = 96)	33%	40%
Private pay (N = 186)	35	42
Insurance other than Blue Cross (N = 165)	35	50
Blue Cross insurance (N = 555)	34	55

* From Avedis Donabedian, "The Quality of Medical Care," in *Medicine in a Changing Society,* ed. Lawrence Corey, Steven Saltman, and Michael Epstein [St. Louis: C. V. Mosby Co., 1972], p. 93. (Data from Sparling, "Measuring Medical Care Quality," *Hospitals* 36 (March 16, 1962), p. 67.)

Beyond this, some type of accountability to professional peers for individual practices is needed, as well as a continuous review of institutional efficiency and correctness in patient care. Peer review is currently receiving much attention. Recent federal legislation has mandated that medical cases paid for by Medicaid and Medicare be reviewed for appropriateness. Under this legislation physician review will be conducted by local doctor groups called Professional Standards Review Organizations. If this system does not operate to the government's satisfaction, then physicians will possibly lose the opportunity for policing their own profession.

There is much agreement among professionals on the necessity of peer review. The form and details of such review are still being debated, and there are possibly many workable alternatives. Effective review committees within hospital settings are to be encouraged, and their scope should include correctness of care, overall physician qualifications, and the responsiveness of the institution to the patient's needs. The danger is not in a too strict control resulting in a repressive atmosphere but rather in the possibility of a review committee developing a lackadaisical approach to review techniques. There must be a determined attempt to identify unnecessary, inadequate, and inappropriate medical care with the basic aim being the improvement of quality through a lessening of human error.

The professional and technical aspects of health care represent only part of the quality problem. The other aspect is the responsiveness of the medical setting to the human needs of the patient. Perhaps more than anything else consumers feel that good quality care involves responding to and treating the whole person.

The increasing specialization of the medical profession has resulted in fragmented, piecemeal services and a lack of continuity in patient care. Good medical care must be organized for the people who receive it, and every effort must be made to overcome the depersonalization currently rampant in many medical settings. No person wants to be treated as a fragmented collection of diseased or partially diseased organs and structures. Being shoveled into a ward and given a number for identification does not alleviate fears or provide personal assurance. Being addressed in a cold, unfeeling manner and treated by a mute retinue of professionals gives the patient no feeling of security or personal value. Oftentimes the fragmentation of services makes it necessary for the patient to travel great distances to receive complete care. Under these conditions receiving good quality health care on a personal basis is at best frustrating and at worst an impossibility. It is essential that efforts be made to make health care not only accessible to the patient but also responsive to his human as well as medical needs. Efforts in this realm have recently been initiated through comprehensive health planning.

Typically, medical practitioners see patients only during a crisis (illness) and consequently do little health-keeping work. Present emphasis is on a continuous comprehensive approach whereby the patient has a close relationship and easy accessibility to the total range of health care. This approach is facilitated by new developments such as prepaid group practice, regional medical centers, neighborhood health clinics, and health maintenance organizations. In every instance the emphasis is on greater coordination of services and on the preventive aspects of health care. Within these new developments special effort is directed toward eliminating the depersonalization in services which so readily detracts from the overall quality of health care.

Better quality medical care is possible. The approaches that will be used will vary according to the dictates of each setting, but it must be kept in mind that the technical aspects of care are only part of the problem. Medical professions must remember that their calling is still one-third science and two-thirds art, and that people identify quality in ways other than technical competence.

THE ORGANIZATIONAL SOLUTION

The problems of inequity, cost, and quality all point to what is perhaps the central problem of health care delivery—organization. Authorities from numerous fields have repeatedly stated that any effective alleviation of the health care crises must involve some alterations in the basic structure of health care organization. A system designed for nineteenth-century medical care is not efficiently operable given the complexity of present-day techniques and problems. As Medicare has demonstrated, pouring additional money into an antiquated system only increases the problems. The magnitude of the complexity in health care may make the reorganization problem seem overwhelming, yet this very complexity offers many avenues of attack through which progress might be made. Proposals for change abound on every side, and many new programs are being tried. Congress is currently debating proposals for a national health insurance program; numerous committees are investigating alternatives to direct federal control of the whole health care industry. The American Medical Association, the drug industry, and numerous professional groups are exploring plans to alleviate the crisis and yet maintain the primacy of democratic principles. Where the organizational issue will lead is difficult to say, but the emergence of some workable alternatives provides clues as to where future health organization might be headed. In the next chapter a few of the innovative approaches to health care delivery will be discussed and an attempt made to assess both the positive and negative aspects of these approaches.

REFERENCES

1. Harold B. Myers, "The Medical-Industrial Complex," *Fortune* (January 1970), p. 90.
2. Basil J. F. Mott, "The Changing Health Care Scene," *Public Administration Review* (September–October 1971), p. 502.
3. Mary W. Herman, "The Poor: Their Medical Needs and the Health Services Available to Them," in *The Annals of the American Academy of Political and Social Science* (January 1972), p. 14.
4. Ibid., pp. 12–21.
5. Raymond S. Duff and August B. Hollingshead, *Sickness and Society* (New York: Harper and Row, 1968), p. 133.
6. Louis H. Henry, "Caring for Our Aged Poor," *The New Republic* (May 22, 1971), p. 19.
7. *Medical Care Costs and Prices—Background Book* (Washington, D.C.: Office of Research and Statistics, U.S. Department of Health, Education, and Welfare, 1972), p. 89.
8. James O. Hepner and Donna M. Hepner, *The Health Strategy Game* (St. Louis: C. V. Mosby Co., 1973), p. 54.
9. Carl M. Cobb, "Solving the Doctor Shortage," *Saturday Review* (August 22, 1970), pp. 24–26.
10. Ibid., p. 25.
11. Ibid.
12. Hepner and Hepner, *The Health Strategy Game,* p. 61.
13. S. G. Kohl, *Perinatal Mortality in New York City: Responsible Factors* (Cambridge, Mass.: Harvard University Press, 1955).
14. Avedis Donabedian, "The Quality of Medical Care," in *Medicine in a Changing Society,* ed. Lawrence Corey, Steven Saltman, and Michael Epstein (St. Louis: C. V. Mosby Co., 1972), p. 97.

SUGGESTED PROJECTS

1. Visit a number of local health care facilities (hospitals, clinics, nursing homes) and interview administrators concerning increasing costs, types of patients, and how they pay for care.

2. With a group of students, prepare a panel discussion on the topic of increasing medical technology, emphasizing both the good and bad aspects of this development.
3. Analyze several health insurance plans and what they actually pay and do not pay for. To do this, you might interview health insurance representatives.

10. Innovations in the Health Field

From efforts to halt the widening gap between reality and expectation in health care have emerged various innovations in health care delivery. This chapter will concentrate on the programs which exemplify basic innovative trends, especially those programs designed to solve the problems identified in the previous chapter. As will become apparent, the problem areas are interrelated: the problem of cost is much entwined with poor organizational structure, and inequity may be greatly affected by the financing procedure. Because of the number of rapid changes in this pioneering area, the emphasis in this chapter will be on current trends and ideologies rather than on an exhaustive listing of specific innovations.

FINANCING MEDICAL CARE

There have always been individuals who could not pay for health care, but the problem has become more acute and widespread as the cost of medical care has increased. At present there are recognized gaps in the quality of care provided to the poor and to the more affluent. Since the advent of Medicare in 1965, costs of health care for the aged have skyrocketed and even the well-to-do find medical costs can be devastating. Consequently, a major renovation in the health care system is in the area of the financing of health care. A major search is underway to find an equitable way of providing adequate health care for *all* people regardless of their ability to pay. The proposals are many but they all seek one end: to provide for the financing of health care for all Americans within the framework of established democratic and free-enterprise principles.

In the early years of this nation, those who could not afford health care were provided for through a charity system generally maintained by private physicians or groups of individuals. With the Great Depression of the nineteen-thirties the number of those who could not pay for health care, as well as for other goods and services, became too large for the charity process. The result was a welfare system initiated by the Social Security Act of 1935 which replaced private charity with public charity. Through this legislation, effort was made to identify people who needed this charity. The resultant "worthy" groups were dependent children, the blind, the aged, and somewhat later in 1950, the permanently and totally disabled. Although the welfare program was not aimed primarily at providing health care, financing of such services did fall under this legislation.

The inherent drawback of the Social Security Act in providing for health needs was its exclusion of many people who could not afford health care but did not fall into the established categories. In addition, it prompted a labeling process which many people found repugnant.

From this beginning in 1935, concern has increased for better and more equitable financing of health care. Both President Roosevelt and President Truman expressed interest in government-backed health insurance, and they were followed by the adamant efforts of Presidents Kennedy and Johnson. In 1960 Kennedy debated the issue of national health insurance for the aged, and in his State of the Union message in 1963 he strongly supported the concept of hospital insurance. Lyndon Johnson also supported these ideas and pushed hard for legislation to provide medical care for the aged under the social security program. The culmination of these efforts was the Medicare Bill, which became law in 1965.

Medicare was a monumental breakthrough in the financing of medical care. As Title XVIII to the Social Security Act, it provides for a major portion of the health expenses of the elderly. It consists of two basic parts. Part A is involuntary and provides a coverage for inpatient hospital service, extended care services (such as nursing homes), home health services, and outpatient diagnostic services. Part B of the law is voluntary, and the person receiving social security benefits must pay a monthly premium to receive this coverage. Under section B, services such as physician consultations, nursing visits, ambulance services, and others not covered under Part A are provided to the individual.

For all its good intentions and pioneering efforts, Medicare has not proven to be a panacea, and there are gaps in its coverage. For example, patients must pay the first 50 dollars of cost under Part B and the first 40 dollars under Part A. In addition, in Part B the patient must pay 20 percent of the total cost. Other stipulations include special limitations on the number of days of extended care and of the care and treatment of mental illness.

The gaps in Medicare are similar to those found in its companion law, Medicaid. Passed in 1965 along with Medicare, this Act is Title XIX of the Social Security law. This program was designed to encourage states, through federal subsidies, to provide care not only to the needy as categorized under the original social security program but also to provide for *any* child or adult who could not afford health care. The long-range objective of Medicaid is to ensure comprehensive health care to all the nation's needy. The most obvious problem with this plan is that it allows each state quite a degree of flexibility in providing for the program. Consequently, some states have provided as many as twenty different services through Medicaid, while in other states the program has been almost nonfunctional.

Both Medicare and Medicaid have proven only partial answers. Out of these pioneering efforts, however, have come new insights and ideas into the financing of health care. Most notably it has become apparent that just changing the financing procedure is not enough. Under Medicare the cost for health care rose dramatically, and data indicate that much of this increase was due to cost-inflating by practitioners who felt that since the government was paying the bill, the individual patient would not be affected by high prices. In other instances there were abuses involving needless hospitalization, treatment, and diagnosis. Regardless of where the blame is placed, the central fact is that changes in the financing procedures must be accompanied by changes in the overall health system.

The payment gaps and other inequities occurring under Medicare and Medicaid, along with financial inequities in the total system, are precipitating some major social and political controversies. That there is a problem is well agreed upon. An acceptable solution, however, is widely debated. A multitude of programs is being proffered but, given the pluralism of viewpoints, disagreement is rampant. For some, government intervention in the financing of health care borders too closely on socialism, and thus one of the major debates is how to provide such financing within democratic principles. One can become lost in the details of each proposal, but the important point is that the problem is now recognized and efforts are underway to alleviate the situation. Some program of government-financed care seems inevitable, but the exact aspects of such a program have yet to be worked out. And whatever plan or plans are finally adopted, it must be realized that these also will have to change as societal needs change.

For the student in community health matters, it is important to understand the problem of financing as only one aspect of community health problems. Solutions to this problem are intricately connected with other aspects of the total health field, and innovations in one area will often affect other problem areas. Consequently, changes in the financing structures must be accompanied by changes in the total structure of health care delivery.

FROM PRIVATE PRACTICE TO HMOs

Reorganization of the health care system is a recurring theme in the present literature. Evidence abounds which indicates that more money or more doctors is not the whole answer: some attempt must be made to restructure the delivery system. Discontent is being voiced over the traditional fee-for-service arrangement in which the physician seems to benefit from the misfortunes of the patient. Many experts further agree that the other problems of quality, equity, and cost can be ameliorated only through reorganization. Consequently, efforts are being made to develop new ways of providing health care. Significant among such developments is the concept of health maintenance organizations (HMO).

The concept of HMOs is grounded in the growing awareness that health care needs have changed while the delivery system has remained the same. Historically, health care has been a personal relationship between the private physician and his patient. The physician was not only a medical healer but family friend and counselor during personal catastrophes. He provided the total spectrum of health care to the patient, offering the best available care in areas as diverse as pediatrics and dermatology. His was an art as much as a science, and sound economic management was not an essential aspect of his life. He often based his fees on the ability of the patient to pay and was well aware that many times he would receive little if any payment for his work.

Slowly, because of the burgeoning medical knowledge, physicians began to realize their inabilities to maintain this omniscient aura. Many began to specialize in order to keep abreast of the latest development in various fields. But, as we have seen, this specialization tended to produce a fragmentation of services which resulted in the treatment of the patient as a series of diseased parts rather than as an integrated whole. In an attempt to move back to the

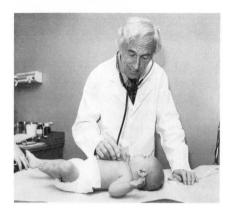
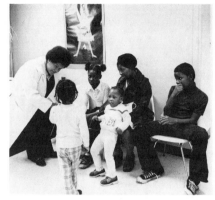

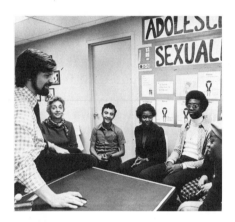
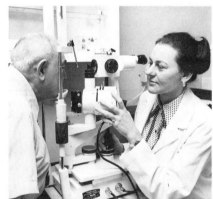

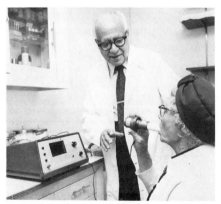
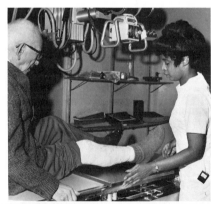

Health maintenance organizations are designed to provide a full range of health care services for all age groups. *(Courtesy of the Health Insurance Plan of Greater New York. Photos by A. Robbins)*

traditional whole-patient approach of the private physician, these specialists began to form group practices. These groups ranged from a very loosely organized situation where the specialists simply shared the same facilities to a highly structured organization where the professionals worked very closely together collaborating on cases, sharing income and expenses, and providing a continuity of comprehensive services for each patient.

Group practice, then, is not a new idea. It has grown out of and is part of the changing nature of the health care system. The concept of the health maintenance organization is an extension of this group practice concept, and rather than being a total break with the past it is simply an evolutionary appendage to an already developed entity. But what are HMOs and how do they function?

An HMO is an organization that provides comprehensive health care to a group of people in return for a predetermined sum of money. The individual pays a fixed amount on a monthly or yearly basis and then receives all of his medical care from this organization. The money may be paid by the individual, by his insurance company, or by the government. By having already paid for it, the patient is not deterred from seeking medical care because of potential costs that might be incurred.

The actual organization of HMOs is quite variable. The large Kaiser Permanente Plan on the West Coast maintains its own hospital system, for example, while the Health Insurance Plan of New York does not. Also, the type of services offered, types of physicians involved, mechanisms for actual delivery of care, and type of patient served may vary. Nonetheless, all HMOs have some basic characteristics which reflect their role in the current health care field: prepayment of medical costs, preventive health maintenance, comprehensive health care, and emphasis on competition and pluralism.

The concept of prepayment is not really new, for it can be found in the traditional insurance programs. Under insurance programs, however, the insurer agrees to pay the cost of health services, while under HMOs the insurer promises to provide the health care. This changes some of the basic incentives of the health system. Generally, every time a patient is treated, the hospital and doctor increase their income. There is thus an incentive to increase services. On the other hand, the income of an HMO is increased when a patient is enrolled; when a service is given it costs the HMO. To maximize its earnings the HMO must hold down its costs. Thus, there is every incentive to treat the patient early, provide preventive care, and use expensive inpatient facilities only when necessary. This economic incentive will also hold down excessive building of facilities and the acquisition of unnecessary equipment. Maintaining empty beds and buying needless equipment are a drain on the money pool of the organization.

There is now an incentive to provide preventive care, since prevention is always cheaper than cure. The physician wishes to keep the individual well so he will need fewer services. This encourages complete health exams, patient education, adequate immunization schedules, and good primary care. HMOs seem to be a beginning toward a true *health* care system with emphasis on prevention rather than cure.

Another positive aspect of HMOs is their emphasis on comprehensive health care. This concept involves the integration of facilities and personnel such that all of a patient's health needs are provided for under one organizational roof. It is a type of one-stop health care for the consumer, and he is guided through the system primarily by one physician who is closest to his needs. This situation makes possible a continuous medical record that can move with the patient and thus encourage continuity of care. There is opportunity for close consultation between physicians on each patient, and peer review becomes more feasible. It is hoped that eventually HMOs will have all elements of care—nursing homes, mental health facilities, dental care—under one organizational arrangement. Thus, when a person walks in the front door, everything he needs in the health area is right there.

The HMO model does not claim to be a solution to all health care problems but rather encourages competition and alternative plans. In providing alternatives to the consumer, HMOs have created a healthy competition in an industry which traditionally has lacked the competitive element. In its support of HMOs, the government is trying to establish nòt a monopoly but rather a varied system which gives the consumer more choice when purchasing medical care. By paying for care in advance, the consumer is freer to choose the kind of health care he wants at the price he wants to pay than he is in an emergency which requires an immediate decision, usually to take the first thing available. Moreover, because the consumer is free "to take it or leave it," HMOs must seriously contend with each other for his business. Competition forces the HMOs to maintain quality in the services and care they provide, for a consumer dissatisfied with one HMO is free to seek care at another.

Yet there are many unanswered questions and doubts about the HMO concept. Those groups that have been in operation for some time, such as Kaiser Permanente and the Health Insurance Plan of New York, provide most of the data on which proponents base their arguments. In truth, however, there has been a paucity of comparative research between the claimed benefits of these programs and other forms of medical practice. For example, one of the vaunted outcomes of the HMO strategy is the fewer number of hospital days per patient as compared to traditional forms of health care. Data from the United States Civil Service Commission on federal employees revealed 60 percent fewer hospital days for those under HMOs as compared with those under indemnity insurance or Blue Cross plans. But it is not clear what mechanisms actually produce this effect. It could be simply that because HMO physicians have fewer hospital beds available to them, they tend to resort less often to hospitalization of their patients.

A further question has been raised concerning the concept of competition working to control abuses in HMO strategy. We suggested that if the consumer has a choice of health plans available to him, he will leave a plan that does not provide quality care. One leading medical sociologist points out, however, that this implies that medical consumers are knowledgeable enough to judge competing forms of care.[1] Such an assumption is often tenuous.

Another consideration that may slant the data in favor of the prepaid, group-practice concept is the type of person enrolled in these groups. Are the consumers who enroll in HMOs more health-conscious and, perhaps, generally healthier individuals? Are they more likely through personal volition to act favorably in regard to their health needs? Such questions are yet to be answered, and it is clear that more research is needed.

The HMO concept should not be viewed as an end to health care problems; rather, it is a beginning which can provide a starting point for the reorganization of the health care system. It is not a flawless model and as yet needs much refinement, but it is a stimulus to further innovations and may provide the insight necessary for the development of a viable health care system in the future.

SURGI-CENTERS: A SOLUTION TO COSTS

It has generally been accepted that surgery means hospitalization. But this idea is being seriously challenged by the recent development of Ambulatory Surgical Treatment Centers. Often referred to a surgi-centers or outpatient surgical centers, these facilities are designed to serve patients who need surgical treatment beyond what can be done in a physician's office but not so complex as to require hospitalization. This allows the patient to have surgery in a comfortable and safe environment with good-quality care, and still to go home the same day.

The surgical center idea got its big boost in 1970 when Dr. John Ford and Dr. Wallace Reed opened their facility in Phoenix, Arizona. Convinced that a significant percentage of hospital surgical cases could be safely and economically performed in an outpatient facility, Drs. Ford and Reed opened their clinic with four goals in mind: "to make the ambulatory patient a matter of greater concern, streamline the delivery of his medical services, reduce the cost of his care, and work for a broadening of his insurance coverage."[2] These goals are the philosophical foundation of the surgicenter concept, and their realization is paramount to its success. From the physical structure to the record-keeping scheme, each part of the clinic is designed to attain the basic goals.

Upon entering the Phoenix facility a patient is briefly interviewed by a receptionist who starts a medical record on the individual. A nurse then takes the patient for any preoperative tests and sees that he is dressed for surgery and made comfortable. During this time the nurse will ask questions and record information concerning his medical history. The patient's temperature will also be taken, and his heart and lungs will be examined by an anesthesiologist. Not until the surgeon is in the facility will the patient be taken to the operating room. Such an arrangement is designed to make the patient feel more comfortable than if he were to wait in the operating room.

In the operating room the patient receives the care of his own physician, plus a qualified anesthesiologist and crew of professional nurses. Following surgery, the patient, according to his own recovery speed, is transferred to a wheelchair and stays seated for a length of time before attempting his own mobility. From entry to exit, the average length of stay is 3½ hours.[3]

The type of surgery possible on such an outpatient basis is determined primarily by the postoperative management necessary. Any procedure that produces postsurgical bleeding or similar complications could not, of course, be performed. But Drs. Ford and Wallace maintain that, with the exception of major surgery involving the abdomen or thorax, almost any surgical operation can be considered for such a facility.

Some patients are not physically right for surgery in such a facility, however. These include individuals with serious heart disease, anemia, or respiratory problems. In addition, individuals who have reservations about the short-stay idea may not be psychologically suited for the experience and should be hospitalized.

To date, the surgi-center concept appears a success. Patients find the "come-and-go surgery" quite convenient, and the personalized care is much appreciated. Consider the difference in lost wages and time between a two-night stay in a hospital and the few hours spent in the ambulatory facility. Moreover, the warm, congenial environment made possible in such a facility provides an atmosphere all too absent in the hospital setting.

But it is cost reduction which has served as the major impetus behind the development of surgical centers, and it is here that the Phoenix facility has most dramatically demonstrated the benefit of the concept (see Tables 10.1 and 10.2). The reasons behind these savings involve the difference in operating expenses between hospitals and surgi-centers. On an inpatient basis, the hospitalized individual must, through his bill, help pay for the "hotel accommodation," "restaurant service," around-the-clock nursing care, and expensive laboratory and medical equipment which are all part of the hospital setting. The surgi-center reduces its operating cost by not needing these things. Further, the savings on an outpatient basis are indicative of more efficient use of personnel and facilities. Dr. Reed of the Phoenix facility has said that four major Phoenix hospitals reduced their operation-room charges for outpatients shortly after his facility was approved by the area health planning council.

TABLE 10.1   The cost of various surgical procedures: surgi-center vs. hospital*

Procedure	Hospital inpatient	Hospital outpatient	Surgi-center (Path. fee inc.)	Savings per case
D. & C.	$265.00		$105.00	$160.00
		$148.90	105.00	43.90
Excision skin lesions	253.00		85.00	168.00
		141.00	85.00	56.00
Bilateral myringotomy	228.33		95.00	133.33
w/tubes		134.31	95.00	39.31
Bilateral inguinal	245.00		150.00	95.00
herniorrhaphy		—0—		
Vasectomy		100.00	85.00	15.00
Excision ganglion	265.00		105.00	160.00
		—0—		
Cystoscopy	295.00		125.00	170.00
		175.00	125.00	50.00
Excision foreign body	210.00		125.00	85.00
		165.00	125.00	40.00
Adenoidectomy and	236.75		95.00	141.75
myringotomy		—0—		
T. & A.	210.00		125.00	85.00
		—0—		

* From Boyden L. Crouch, John L. Ford, and Wallace A. Reed, "The Surgical Center: Concept, Care, and Cost in Freestanding Facility," *Hospital Topics* (December 1971).

Still, the Phoenix surgi-center cost for comparable procedures averaged 130 dollars less than the hospital costs.[4]

Surgi-centers do seem successful, and the savings in cost appear a real breakthrough. Nonetheless, there are some critics, and some officials have reservations about these facilities. First, the concept of a "free-standing" clinic is seen as a threat by the medical establishment. A free-standing clinic is not part of a hospital complex and is not subject to administrative rule of any other medical facility. Hospitals, as might be expected, view such facilities as serious competitors for the health care dollars. Some critics claim that these clinics duplicate facilities and could prove more economical in the long run if they were part of the hospital, thereby having the advantages of extant facilities, institutional purchasing power, and savings on staff. But proponents of the surgical centers see their work not as fragmentation but as a wise division of labor. Their analogy is that of a large automobile manufacturer subcontracting

TABLE 10.2   Estimated savings for surgi-center patients in first 3,000 cases*

Procedure	# Cases in first 3,000	# Instead of hospital outpatient	# Instead of hospital inpatient	Savings per case	Total savings
D. & C.					
(only diagnostic)	565	57		$ 43.90	$ 2,502.30
			508	160.00	81,280.00
Excision skin	238	24		56.00	1,344.00
lesions			214	168.00	35,952.00
Bilateral myringotomy w/tubes	228	23		39.31	904.13
			205	133.33	27,332.65
Bilateral inguinal herniorrhaphy	174		174	95.00	16,530.00
Vasectomy	154	154		15.00	2,310.00
Excision ganglion	88		88	160.00	14,080.00
Cystoscopy	75	8		50.00	400.00
			67	170.00	11,390.00
Excision foreign body	58	6		40.00	240.00
			52	85.00	4,420.00
Adenoidectomy and myringotomy	54		54	141.75	7,654.50
T. & A.	43		43	85.00	3,555.00
Other	1,323	132		28.31	3,736.92
			1,191	143.91	171,396.81
	3,000	404	2,596		$385,028.31

* From Boyden L. Crouch, John L. Ford, and Wallace A. Reed, "The Surgical Center: Concept, Care, and Cost in Freestanding Facility," *Hospital Topics* (December 1971).

certain parts to smaller companies which can turn out the needed product more efficiently and economically. In addition, the proponents feel that hospitals want to impose regulations and control which in many instances may be unrealistic for the facility.

Another charge against surgical centers is that they do not have the intensive care facilities or monitoring equipment available in large hospitals to meet emergencies. The answer to this criticism is that the surgical-center concept stresses transfer agreements with nearby hospitals so that any time an emergency does arise the patient can expeditiously be transferred to the hospital. Secondly, it is pointed out by the founders of the Phoenix surgi-center that during the first 17 months of operation, there has never been a need to take advantage of the transfer agreement with the local hospitals.

Barring criticisms about such surgical centers, the idea seems to be gaining in momentum. The Phoenix facility has now been in operation for several years and its success has spawned other such clinics across the country.

The surgical-center concept is an innovation. It provides a savings in cost at a time when health care costs are ballooning. The major concern is now how well it, along with other health care innovations, will mesh into the total health care scheme. Is it another example of fragmentation, or is it the type of facility that will work well into a comprehensive health care delivery system? Future experience can be the only answer.

COMPREHENSIVE HEALTH PLANNING: TOWARD BETTER ORGANIZATION

In 1966 Congress passed the Comprehensive Health Planning and Public Health Services Act. The intent of this legislation, later known as the Partnership for Health Act, was the establishment of statewide and local area comprehensive health planning agencies. These agencies were to be responsible for health planning that involved all sectors of the community, with emphasis on coordination between consumers and providers. Further, the Act stressed that the federal government did not wish to dominate or centralize the planning process, but wished to place major responsibility with the states and the local community. To ensure this it stipulated that a council, composed of volunteers from the local health services and representative consumers from the local area, be formed to decide all matters of policy in the agency. This planning mechanism attempts to bring the community together to identify problems, plan solutions, and overcome the haphazard design and implementation characteristic of the past.

Under this legislation federal funds are made available to the state and local areas for planning purposes. This money may be given in the form of a grant for a special project or for the general purpose of financing a state planning agency.

Within the planning framework each state is to establish a single administrative body to be known as the "a" agency which will oversee all comprehensive health planning activities within the state. In addition, the state must appoint an advisory state health planning council and develop an encompassing statewide plan which pinpoints the state and local activities to be funded by federal monies.

At local and areawide levels, agencies are to be developed to undertake both comprehensive planning and project development for their area. Known as "b" agencies, these groups serve as the real key in the planning process, for they involve the consumers and can identify the felt needs of the community. In this coordinated effort, the state agency serves as a review group which constructively evaluates the efforts undertaken by local "b" planning groups.

Under the concept of comprehensive health planning, special

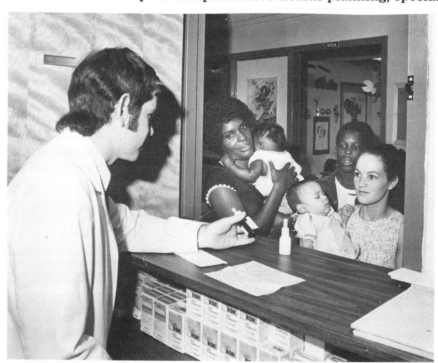

In one effort to centralize health care services, Beth Israel Medical Center in New York City set up a community-oriented pediatrics pharmacy on its pediatrics outpatient floor so that parents may pick up medicine for their children without the inconvenience of leaving the immediate area. *(Courtesy of Beth Israel Medical Center)*

emphasis is placed on improving health planning and health services at the community level. Although the final approval for a project rests with the state agency, responsibility for the basic planning lies with the local, areawide group.

To date, most of the effort has focused on the development of standards and guidelines by the state and local agencies to be used in planning new facilities (such as hospitals and clinics) and renovating or relocating existing ones. In some states the state agencies have gained considerable power through legislation which requires that a proposed change of an existing facility or the building of a new one meet criteria in accordance with the needs of the community to be affected. The first such law, known as Certification of Need Law, was passed in New York in 1966. Under this law, the state commissioner of health as well as the state and local hospital planning councils must give their approval before any private or public hospital may be built. Their combined approval is referred to as a "certificate of need." Such legislation ensures the controlled growth of the health care industry and maximum efficiency in meeting the health needs of the population. It helps to give some power to the planning process and forces some control on the proliferation of unwarranted or poorly planned facilities.

Comprehensive health planning is representative of an attempt to overcome the poor planning that plagues the delivery of health care in this country. It attempts this through better coordination of federal, state, and local efforts and more local and state control in the actual planning of health policies and programs. In its efforts to promote better planning, CHP has concentrated on community groups and has emphasized the role of the consumer in the planning process. A majority of the membership of the state planning councils must be composed of consumer representatives. In addition, consumers must be present in the development and operation of the projects receiving funds through CHP grants. It is this emphasis on consumer participation which marks one of the real insights and positive aspects of comprehensive health planning.

Representative as it is of a trend toward better planning, CHP may prove more a transient beginning than a stable part of the health field. Its importance, however, is in its concepts, and these may prove valuable as a stimulus for future organizational innovations.

CONSUMERISM: A NEW FORCE IN THE HEALTH FIELD

Traditionally, the health care consumer has occupied a spectator's role in the health care arena, with little opportunity to be involved in the decisions which affect the organization and delivery of the care that he receives. Awed by medical science and often intimidated by its practitioners, the consumer has seldom been approached for input as to the gaps he felt in the health care system or the kinds of needs he had which were not being met. But this situation is rapidly changing. In fact, "consumerism" in the health field is a rapidly growing reality.

The role of the consumer got a big boost with the Comprehensive Health Planning Law of 1966. As previously stated, this law mandated consumer representation on all planning groups, and it called for active consumer participation in the development and operation of projects supported by CHP funds. It further stipulated that the consumer representatives should be so chosen as to reflect a broad spectrum of geographic and socioeconomic groups. This act opened new avenues for consumer influence in the formulation and implementation of community health policy.

Since the consumer himself is the one closest to his health problems, he is in a better position than the professional, if not to evaluate them and determine their solutions, at least to recognize where they exist and decide their relative priority. The health professional, accustomed to relying primarily on his own judgments in health matters, will increasingly find consumer action in and scrutiny of the programs he designs. Such scrutiny will, it is hoped, provide a climate in which programs that best meet the needs of the consumer can be pursued. There is no better indicator of a program's value than if it meets the health needs of the consumer as identified by *both* the consumer and the professional.

The Comprehensive Health Planning Law is, then, a prime example of the recognition of the health consumer as a viable force in the planning of health care. But in the actual participation in a health program, the consumer movement has also received major support from the neighborhood health center concept.

The neighborhood health center idea is an outgrowth of the Economic Opportunity Act of 1964. This antipoverty legislation sought ways in which the federal government could most effectively assist local communities in their efforts to eradicate poverty. It soon became apparent to individuals working in the local communities that health needs were inextricably linked to the total poverty complex. It was obvious that educational improvements meant nothing to children whose physical problems made learning impossible. Consequently, pressure was brought to bear on the Office of Economic Opportunity (OEO) to make funds available to provide for more efficient health care for the poor.

At this same time many realized that the traditional delivery mechanisms were failing the poor and that any hope for better health care would necessitate fundamental changes in the arrangements for organizing and delivering health services. Thus OEO workers decided to devote some research and demonstration funds to projects that would point to possible solutions to this organizational problem. Through discussions, input from health professionals, and close work with officials at all levels, there developed the basic outlines of what was to become known as the neighborhood health center. The basic characteristics of this facility were envisaged as follows:

1. Focus on the needs of the poor
2. A one-door facility, readily accessible in terms of time and place, in which all ambulatory health services are made available
3. Intensive participation by and involvement of the population to be served, both as policy-makers and as employees
4. Full integration of and with existing sources of services and funds
5. Assurance of personalized, high-quality care and professional staff of the highest caliber
6. Close coordination with other community resources
7. Sponsorship by a wide variety of public and private auspices.[5]

The idea received a good response, and by the summer of 1966 eight demonstration neighborhood health centers had been approved. The concept of providing good-quality care to the poor in a convenient and familiar setting seemed a tenable solution to the inequities of health care endured by the poor. In addition, never before had the consumer been so involved in the actual health care process. It is in this new involvement of the consumer that much of the positive value of the neighborhood health center concept can be found.

The role of the consumer in these centers was twofold. First, the consumers were given a major role in planning and, eventually, in actual policy-making. In the early days of their development, the neighborhood health centers were provider-dominated and consumers were often called to serve after the basic proposal had been submitted for governmental support. This led to alienation of the consumer, and it became readily apparent that consumers and providers should work together in the initiation, planning, and implementation of the program. The consumer thus became recognized as a major voice in the basic policy-making decisions of the health facility.

Secondly, the consumers in neighborhood health centers often

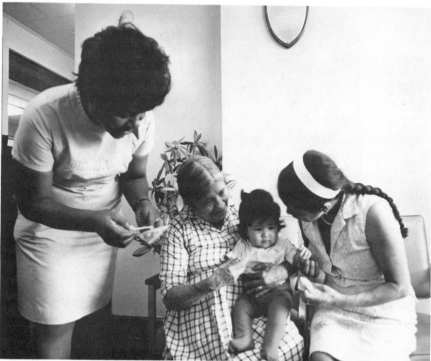

A Spanish-speaking public health nurse explains the renewal process of the Medicaid card to members of a Mexican-American family. The grandmother, mother, and her daughter are all cared for by this neighborhood health center. *(Courtesy of the Bureau of Human Resources Development, National Institutes of Health)*

function as actual health workers. In this instance local residents are trained as health workers to meet a multitude of needs, many of which involve various aspects of home nursing. The recruitment, training, and employment of local residents gives the neighborhood health center a much closer tie with the population being served and thus breaks down many social barriers that often exist between providers and consumers of health care.

This role of the consumer is illustrated in the family health worker program in the Martin Luther King Neighborhood Health Center in New York. Although this program is no longer in existence, it provides an excellent example of the kinds of duties and functions of the consumer health worker that are carried out in other neighborhood centers. The following description of the program was given by Dr. Harold Wise, project director of the Martin Luther King center.

The family health worker's base is the health center, but much of her time is involved in making home visits in the community. She is the third member of the medical team, along with the physician and the public health nurse. She is assigned to 40 to 60 families. Her day-to-day supervision comes from the public health nurse on her team; continuing inservice training comes from a family health worker supervisor—a public health nurse whose prime assignment is training.

Daily activities of the family health worker include a variety of health education, patient care, and social advocacy activities. She instructs the new mother how to bathe and feed the baby, and is alert to household hazards such as fire traps and broken paint on walls. In her training strong emphasis is placed on patient education, case finding, the preventive aspects of medical care, and the emotional factors influencing illness.

Her patient care activities include checking blood pressure and pulse (as on a known hypertensive patient recently discharged from the hospital); instructing relatives of bedbound patients (bathing, skin care, changing dressings, irrigating catheters, giving enemas), carrying out the exercises prescribed by a physiatrist; checking whether a new diabetic patient understands how to check his urine and is following his diet. . . .

During the course of her home visits the family health worker deals with a variety of social and environmental problems. She assists a patient with heart disease to obtain a telephone through the Welfare Department, or to obtain more suitable, low-income housing for a large young family.[6]

The neighborhood health center is an innovation, and like many innovations its major value may lie in the promotion of its basic concepts rather than its endurance as a permanent fixture in the health care system. The involvement of the consumer in the policy-making and actual delivery of health care may prove to have a long-lasting effect on health care delivery. Making health facilities more responsive to the needs of the consumer rather than organizing them for the convenience of the provider is a major trend of the future. What the future of neighborhood health centers will be is difficult to predict. Recently, their federal funding has been drastically reduced. Regardless of their actual future, however, their impact as originators of change is significant.

The expansion of the role of the consumer in health matters has been accompanied by an increasing responsibility on the part of the individual for his own health. As a consequence, growing emphasis is being placed on health education for the consumer. Informed consumers are of paramount importance to a health system dedicated to comprehensive health care and emphasizing prevention and health maintenance, and effective health education of the general public is required to develop such consumers. Health information must be carried in the media, taught in schools, provided in the community, emphasized in industry, and provided wherever an audience is found which needs and is receptive to health education. The ultimate responsibility for the health of the individual lies, of course, with the individual. To assume his responsibility fully, however, the individual must be well informed on health matters. And it is on the foundation of responsible and educated citizens that the success of any national, comprehensive health care system rests.

This emphasis on public health information is new in scope rather than concept, for public health officials have always seen education as part of their services. The really new innovation in consumer education involves the recognition that the doctor and medical care setting have a high potential as providers of health education. There is a growing list of ailments that can be effectively managed by proper medication, diet, life style, and so on. Diabetes, arthritis, heart disease, blood problems, and many dietary ailments can be adequately controlled. But the effectiveness of the medical technique often depends on the knowledge and cooperation of the patient who must follow the physician's recommendations. Awareness of this necessity of the patient's cooperation has led to a major trend in health care delivery known as patient education.

With emphasis again on the consumer, patient education is yet another attempt to make the individual health consumer a responsible member of the overall health care team. Patient education provides educational experiences planned and implemented for the patient by the health professionals (nurses, physicians, health educators, and administrators) who are responsible for his well-being. The educational experience can be a workshop, a one-day meeting, a series of lectures or demonstrations, or a personal conference with a patient; it may involve one patient or several. Often the family of a patient will be given information and advice concerning the patient's problem and how best to aid him in the management of his illness.

The emphasis in these programs is on the utilization of the physician-hospital setting to implement the educational process. An example of such a program is the one that was conducted at St. Peter's General Hospital in New Brunswick, New Jersey. At this hospital a team of health professionals established an educational program for 50 outpatients with congestive heart failure. The educational team used individual conferences in the clinic and in the home, as well as sessions with groups of patients. By means of three control groups of comparable patients, it was found that the study group showed increases in knowledge concerning their problem, the medication used, and the diet necessary for control of the ailment. Further data analysis showed that the study group had fewer hospital admissions and shorter stays.[7]

Another program conducted at the Presbyterian Hospital in Newark, New Jersey, concentrated on education for mastectomy patients. The program was directed at postsurgery inpatients and was designed to explain exercises and prosthetic devices and to inform the patient of appropriate agencies to contact for assistance. In addition, the program sought to establish a group of patients who had undergone this surgery and would meet regularly to discuss problems of mutual interest. Eventually there were monthly group meetings open not only to patients from the Presbyterian Hospital, but to mastectomy patients from all the hospitals in the Newark area.[8]

This concept of patient education is rapidly gaining wide acceptance, and already programs for diabetics, cancer victims, and persons with heart ailments can be found in many hospitals. In light of the current emphasis on the knowledgeable consumer it is a laudable and timely innovation. Further, with the push for compre-

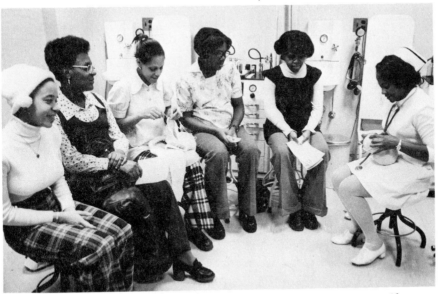

The hospital setting is increasingly being used for patient education programs. Above, an RN at the United Hospitals Medical Center in Newark, New Jersey, demonstrates the birth of a baby by use of a model to expectant mothers who come to the center's prenatal clinic. *(Courtesy of the United Hospitals Medical Center)*

hensive health care there is an ever-growing need for coordination between treatment and teaching. The uninformed patient is in a poor position both to assess his health needs and to carry through with physician recommendations once his problem is diagnosed. A beginning toward comprehensive health is the acceptance of the premise that a patient has the right to know not only the nature of his health problem but also the community resources available to help him with it and methods for the personal management of his condition so as to prevent or minimize future problems and complications.

The active involvement of the consumer in his own health care further reinforces the new role of the health consumer. More emphasis is being placed on education, and the days when the health consumer was an awe-struck mute in the presence of medical science are passing rapidly. Responsible for a health bill of close to 80 billion dollars, he is an emerging active force in the health care field, and the consumer movement may prove to be one of the most significant changes occurring in American health care.

MEDICAL MANPOWER: MEETING THE DEMAND

In the previous chapter some consideration was given to the shortage of physicians as part of the current dilemma in health care delivery. Two basic solutions to this problem were reviewed: increase the number of physicians, or increase the productivity of physicians. It was further stated that although both solutions should be pursued, the latter solution seemed more feasible for the immediate future. Consequently, most of the efforts to alleviate the manpower shortage involve innovations in the utilization of health manpower and the development of new specialties to enhance the productivity of the medical professions.

Chief among these innovations to meet the needs for medical manpower is the training of physician assistants. In any setting where the physician functions, of course, all the ancillary personnel (nurses, technicians, and so on) assist the physician. But the title of physician assistant refers to an individual with specialized training which enables him or her to perform duties previously assigned solely to the physician. With physicians in many specialty areas finding increased demands on their time, the physician assistant can be delegated specific duties, functions, and responsibilities which will release the physician for more specialized tasks.

The programs to train physician assistants vary according to the type of student being trained and to the specialty area in which the person is being prepared. In many instances the program will give advanced training to individuals already experienced in the health program. For example, many programs take nurses and give them additional training; in other instances, such as the Medex program discussed in the previous chapter, medical corpsmen are enrolled in an intensive training program followed by a period of "field" experience working under the supervision of a physician.

At the University of Colorado there is a program to train pediatric nurse-practitioners. The enrolling student must have a BS degree in nursing prior to entering the program. The training period involves four months of intensive theory and practice in pediatrics during which the nurse becomes proficient in performing complete physical exams, including using instruments such as the stethoscope and other necessary examining equipment. The nurse also is schooled in various aspects of parent-child relationships, physical and psychosocial development, infant nutrition, immunization procedures and techniques on counseling with parents. Following his or her training period, the pediatric nurse-practitioner works in the offices of pediatricians or in field-stations in low-income urban and rural areas.

In their work these nurses perform a broad range of child-care

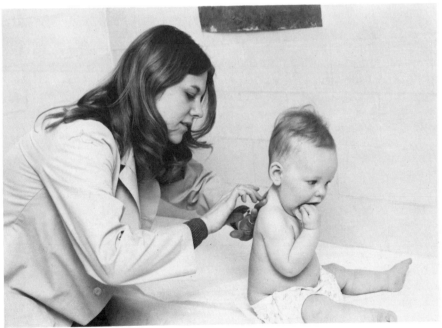

Well-baby examinations are part of the work of the child health associate at the University of Colorado. *(Courtesy of the University of Colorado Medical Center)*

duties that previously would have taken up a physician's time. Routine checkups of infants and older children, instruction on aspects of child care to young mothers, performance of screening tests, administering immunizations, and management of minor disorders all fall under the professional skill of the pediatric nurse-practitioner. Thus, while utilizing their high level of professional skill, these nurses allow for the more effective and judicious use of the specialist's skills. When problems beyond his scope arise, the nurse refers them to the physician's expertise, and there is a close coordination and continuity of care provided through the two cooperating professionals.

In evaluating the competence and overall effectiveness of these pediatric nurse-practitioners, researchers have found very positive responses. Out of some 2,700 patient visits to an urban neighborhood child health station, 71 percent were handled by the nurse-practitioner and another 11 percent were managed with only telephone consultation with the pediatrician. Ninety-four percent of parents surveyed expressed their satisfaction with combined services of pediatrician and pediatric nurse-practitioner. Further, it was found that pediatricians who have nurse-practitioners as associates in their practice have one-third more time for patient care and various other professional duties.[9]

Whereas the pediatric nurse-practitioner and Medex programs utilize health professionals in short-term training, there are also longer-term programs designed to train people for new medical specialties which involve about five years of training. These programs generally take people with two years of college premedical studies or some practical experience, such as corpsmen, and give them an additional year of academic training plus one year of clinical training and one year of internship.

Typical of such a program is the one at Duke University in Durham, North Carolina. There the physician's associate program requires nine months of academic work followed by fifteen months of clinical practice. The student's training prepares him for work with either general or specialist physicians, and emphasis is placed on his assuming many of the routine tasks traditionally performed by the physician.

The University of Colorado has a similar program, known as the Child Health Associate Program, which trains health professionals to work with physicians in giving diagnostic, preventive, and therapeutic services to children. Students in the program must have completed at least two years of work in an undergraduate college. The student then is given a two-year course of instruction followed by a one-year internship. Following this training and the successful

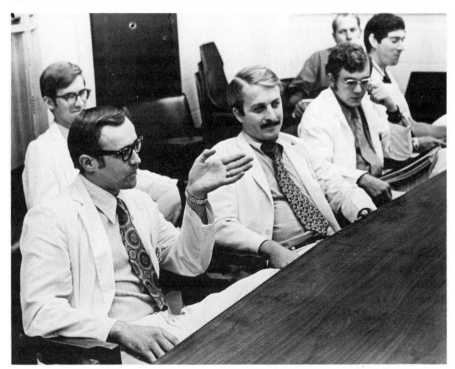

The physician's associate program at Duke University, requiring two years of post-college training both inside and outside the classroom, is one of the longer-term programs designed to train specialized health professionals. *(Courtesy of Duke University Medical Center)*

completion of an examination by the State Board of Medical Examiners, the child health associate will be able to assume the supervision of health care for most well children and many of those who are injured or sick.

These examples are only a few of the beginning schemes to increase physician productivity through the use of physician assistants. Judging from the amount of literature on the topic and the positive data gathered by researchers, the concept seems to have a definite future in the health care field. For not only will the use of these assistants allow the physician more time to employ his special talents where they are most needed, it also will mean that many who were not receiving care at all will now have access to it and those who had been receiving some medical attention will get better service and at less rapidly rising costs.

The goal of increasing the physician's productivity through the use of the physician assistant does not deny the need to increase the number of trained physicians. Medical schools are beginning to expand across the nation, and their enrollments are being increased to their highest level. Between 1965 and 1971 medical schools increased their entering class size from 8,759 to 12,361. Moreover, federal grants are being offered to bolster the manpower output of these schools, thus prompting the further development of facilities. Thus, the training of paramedical personnel is one aid in overcoming the medical manpower shortage, but it does not negate the need for increasing the education and training of more physicians.

In addition to the training of more physicians and of such paraprofessionals as physician assistants, the manpower problem is also being attacked through the use of automation. Computers especially are beginning to emerge as real boons to manpower productivity. They have, for example, a potential use in patient diagnosis. By giving the computer information on a patient's symptoms along with laboratory and X-ray results, the physician can estimate the probability of his patient's having a certain disease, and thus he has a more scientific basis for his decisions. Similarly, computers have proven useful in multiphasic screening. In multiphasic screening the patient receives a variety of tests, and the information from

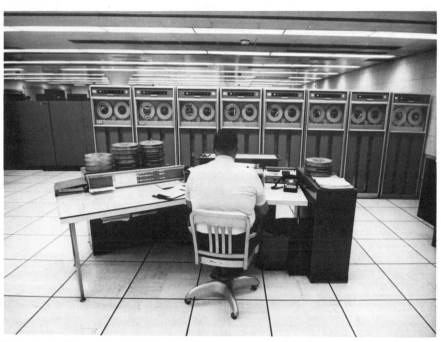

Not only do the computers provide mathematical and statistical analyses, they also make predictions. Plugged into the operating table, they can offer the surgeon a prognosis while he is still at the patient's side. Above is shown the data-processing equipment used to aid medical research at the National Institutes of Health. *(Courtesy of the World Health Organization)*

them is scanned for possible abnormalities. Using the computer it is possible to conduct an elaborate and thorough examination with minimal manpower output. The multiphasic computerized unit can conduct chemical and electronic tests, and because it is automated, both the tests and central data are processed rapidly.

The actual use of computers in medicine is in its infancy, but the possibilities seem staggering. The current uses of computers range from collecting, organizing, and retrieving medical data to monitoring intensive care units to establishing a record of deceased organ donors to match with potential organ recipients.[10] In other instances computer technology has been used to develop complete information retrieval systems for hospital pharmacies and for the programming of automatic food carts which can also be used to deliver linens and medical supplies. In each case, there are considerable savings of manpower through the use of this technology.

Some real efforts are now being made to relieve the shortage of medical manpower. The training of more physicians and development of new paramedical specialties are both being pursued. The latter offers the hope of releasing the more specialized physician from tasks which formerly took much of his time. For the very near future the trend appears to be special, short-term training for individuals already in the health care field. These programs can provide much needed personnel relatively quickly. Longer-range programs such as the Child Health Associate Program in Colorado offer some exciting possibilities, but it will be a few years before such programs can add a significant number of professionals to the health care field.

Although automation, computers, and other technological advances do offer the possibility of manpower savings, there are some problems at this time, including costs and the training of specialists to maintain the technology. It must also be remembered that the technology is only part of a larger system, and if the medical personnel and administrative structure are not functioning well, the technology will not be effective.

SUMMARY

Americans have experienced a major gap between their expectations and the reality of the health care they receive. To bridge this gap, a number of innovations have recently appeared. The examples offered in this chapter are indicative of some of the broad trends in overcoming the problem, and though the specific examples may be short-lived, it must be emphasized that their importance often lies more in their basic underlying concepts than in the duration of their structural existence. The future of certain neighborhood health centers may be in doubt, for example, but their basic principles are indicative of emerging trends in the health field.

No attempt has been made to develop an exhaustive list of innovations; rather, the discussions have concentrated on those general areas in which basic innovations are being pursued. In general, current innovations in the health field fall into the following categories:

1. Innovations in organization and delivery (HMOs, surgicenters)
2. New methods and emphasis on training health manpower
3. The application of technology to tasks and activities of medical personnel
4. Comprehensive health planning and administrative innovations designed to involve the consumer
5. New methods of financing health care.

REFERENCES

1. David Mechanic, *Public Expectations and Health Care: Essays on the Changing Organization of Health Services* (New York: John Wiley and Sons, Inc., 1972), p. 109.
2. *American Medical News,* "Come-and-Go Surgery Sparks Controversy," (November 29, 1971), p. 8.
3. Boyden L. Crouch, John L. Ford, and Wallace A. Reed, "The Surgical Center: Concept, Care, Cost in Freestanding Facility," *Hospital Topics* (December 1971).
4. *American Medical News,* Ibid., p. 7.
5. Lisbeth Bamberger Schorr, "The Neighborhood Health Center—Background and Current Issues," in *Medicine in a Changing Society,* ed. Lawrence Corey, Steven Saltman, and Michael Epstein (St. Louis: C. V. Mosby Co., 1972), p. 140.
6. Ibid., pp. 143–144.
7. Daniel Sullivan, ed., *Health Education Report* (March–April 1974), p. 6.
8. Florence B. Fiori, Marguerite de la Vega, Mary J. Vaccaro, "Health Education in a Hospital Setting: Report of a Public Health Service Project in Newark, New Jersey," in *Health Education Monographs,* ed. Ruth F. Richards and Howard Kalmer (Thorofare, N.J.: Charles B. Slack, Inc., Spring 1974), p. 16–17.
9. Henry K. Silver and James A. Hecker, "The Pediatric Nurse Practitioner and the Child Health Associate: New Types of

Health Professionals," *Journal of Medical Education,* 45 (March 1970): 172–173.

10. James O. Hepner and Donna M. Hepner, *The Health Strategy Game* (St. Louis: C. V. Mosby Co., 1973), p. 255.

SUGGESTED PROJECTS

1. With a panel of students, do an in-depth study of national health insurance. Interview a number of physicians, insurance representatives, and hospital administrators to get their feelings about such a program, and then give a class presentation on the pertinent issues surrounding the idea of national health insurance.
2. Make a survey of local health facilities to determine if there are any patient education programs in existence. Where such programs exist, prepare a class presentation on the programs.
3. Prepare an analysis of the evolution of the physician's role in American society. Starting with the early days of this country, review the role of the physician and his impact on the patient. Also discuss the concept that medicine is an art as much as a science.
4. If there is a Comprehensive Health Planning group in the local area, attend several of its meetings to learn about its purpose and role in the community.
5. Discuss the concept of consumerism in health care. Have you or your family had any experiences that reflect consumer input (or lack thereof) into the health care field?

INDEX